Insulin Resistance And Pcos Cookbook

"the new complete guide treat, prevent insulin resistance and PCOS with natural remedies"

Charles Thompson

Copyright© 2020by Charles Thompson

Contents

Insulin Resistance Diet Plan 6

Introduction 6

Chapter 1: What is insulin resistance..................................7

Causes 7

Symptoms 8

Risks and complications 10

Treatments 11

Diagnosis and exams 14

Chapter 2: Insulin resistance prevention 15

How can food help? 15

Physical activity 19

Lifestyle 21

Chapter 3: Breakfast 23

Chapter 4: Appetizers and Snacks 39

Chapter 5: Meat 59

Chapter 6: Fish & Seafood 74

Chapter 7: Unique dishes 90

Chapter 8: Side Dish 105

Chapter 9: Dessert 118

Chapter 10: Sauces & Condiment 131

Conclusion 144

PCOS Cookbook 145

Introduction 146

Chapter 1: What is PCOS? 147

    Types of PCOS 147

    Causes 149

    Symptoms 151

    PCOS diagnosis.. 153

Chapter 2: Treatments, risks and complications 155

    Treatments... 155

    Risks and complications 160

Chapter 2: PCOS and diet................................... 162

    Foods to eat 162

    Foods to avoid.. 163

    Example meal plan.................................... 163

Chapter 3: Breakfast 174

Chapter 4: Snack, Side, Appetizers 186

Chapter 5: Meat.. 200

Chapter 6: Fish & Seafood 215

Chapter 7 : Soup & Salad 230

Chapter 8: Dessert 245

Chapter 9: Sauces & Condiments 259

Conclusion... 273

Insulin Resistance Diet Plan

Introduction

Insulin was discovered in 1921 by the Englishman John James Macleod and the Canadian Frederick Grant Bating, Nobel prize for medicine in 1923. Insulin is a hormone produced by the pancreas. The role of insulin is to allow the body's cells to incorporate glucose to be used as fuel or stored as body fat. Insulin has multiple functions: it facilitates the passage of glucose from the blood to the cells and therefore has an action to lower blood sugar, facilitates the passage of amino acids in the blood, stimulates the use of glucose and fatty acids as energy production, facilitates the passage of potassium inside the cells and stimulates the endogenous production of cholesterol. When glucose is not properly incorporated, it is more likely to accumulate in the blood and lead to too high blood sugar levels. The body then becomes insulin resistant and tries to cope with the problem by producing larger quantities. The pancreas' excessive work causes a functional decline of the cells used for the production of insulin, and one can speak for all effects of type II diabetes mellitus. Therefore insulin resistance precedes, even a few years, the appearance of diabetes mellitus. If left untreated, insulin resistance can also lead to other complications, including heart, kidney, and liver problems. So it is important to change your diet associated with a correct lifestyle completely. In this guide, you will find everything you need to know about insulin resistance, a healthy diet, and many useful tips to change your lifestyle.

Chapter 1: What is insulin resistance

Insulin resistance is a condition that arises when the body's cells have poor insulin sensitivity. This inability of the cells means that glucose is not absorbed. Consequently, the prolongation of glucose in the blood leads to increased blood glucose levels and an accumulation of insulin in the body as it is not forfeited in the cells. When there is excessive insulin production by the pancreas in the case of a wrong diet, the cellular insulin receptors are constantly stimulated by the hormone. Consequently, the cell finds itself absorbing more sugar than necessary.

Causes

Over the course of life, due to congenital or acquired factors, cells may become less sensitive to insulin; in these cases, we speak of insulin resistance. The pancreas tries to compensate for the reduced cell sensitivity by increasing the synthesis and release of the hormone. When this condition becomes chronic, the overload of the pancreas and the negative effects of hyperinsulinemia itself on cellular sensitivity, cause a functional decline of the cells used for insulin production and the appearance of hyperglycemia.

The main causes of insulin resistance are listed below:
- Genetic defects: In some cases, the insulin receptor's genetic defects do not work well because it is not formed correctly.
- Poor nutrition: High-calorie diet, with high sugar content or rich in carbohydrates.

- Sedentary life: Lack of exercise and consequent weight gain are among the most common causes of insulin resistance.
- Immunology: pathologies of the immune system that cause the development of autoantibodies that are against the insulin receptor can cause insulin resistance.
- Hormones: excessive production of growth hormones hinders the insulin receptor with the hormone and consequently causes a lower receptor efficiency.
- Pharmacy: those who make extensive use of corticosteroids can be subject to insulin resistance as the values of hormones that are enemies of insulin are increased.
- Being obese or overweight: In particular, the waist circumference width, i.e., the amount of abdominal fat, is decisive. Furthermore, excess fat in the abdominal area is more associated with cardiovascular diseases, especially in the presence of high cholesterol.
- Hypertriglyceridemia or the values of triglycerides in the blood too high.
- Low HDL cholesterol levels. HDL cholesterol is considered good, as it reduces the chances of cardiovascular disease. On the contrary, having it low increases the risk of these pathologies insulin resistance
- Having high levels of stress

Symptoms

Initially, insulin resistance does not show any symptoms. Initially, the resistance of the cells is compensated by the increased production of insulin. Symptoms begin to appear only when they lead to side effects such as higher blood sugar levels. When compensation no longer occurs, and a hyperglycemic condition occurs, the following symptoms may occur:

- Weight gain

Insulin resistance causes an alteration of fatty acids. Fatty acids are increased in the body, which comes from excess glucose in the body. The accumulation of fatty acids leads to weight gain and are mainly deposited by the abdominal part. Excess fats also risk depositing on the liver, risking liver steatosis. At the level of the arteries, the greater amount of fatty acids leads to a high risk of arteriosclerosis.

- Drowsiness and tiredness

In most cases, drowsiness and fatigue are the first symptoms that lead to insulin resistance. They are easy to find symptoms, along with difficulty concentrating.

- A greater sense of hunger

Hunger is another very tangible symptom. Hunger caused by insulin resistance is often a nervous hunger. Nervous hunger leads to binges and many snacks throughout the day, with an excessive intake of calories. All this leads to excessive insulin production.

- High levels of bad LDL cholesterol

LDL cholesterol is considered "bad" and is basically the fat in the blood. This fat circulates in the body and leads to a high risk of heart attack, stroke, and arteriosclerosis.

- High pressure

Blood pressure is due to the heart's pulse, which normally generates enough thrust to make blood flow throughout the body. With high blood pressure, this thrust is higher than the normal body needs. Hypertension leads to a high risk of heart attack, stroke, Parkinson's disease, and cerebral ischemia.

Risks and complications

As previously explained, in the condition of insulin resistance, the liver cells do not respond adequately to insulin stimulation. Thus, the cells are no longer able to correctly and quickly absorb glucose. The sugars remain in the bloodstream, causing hyperglycemia, a situation that can lead to prediabetes, diabetes, and other ailments. Risks and complications can be:

- Heart disease

For example, pathologies affecting the heart's valves, congenital malformations, and all those diseases that can alter the functioning of the heart pump belong to the category of heart disease.

- Stroke

The term stroke and its numerous synonyms indicate a loss of brain function, caused by an insufficient supply of blood to a more or less extensive area of the organ. Without this fundamental blood supply, brain tissue begins to die from the absence of oxygen and nutrients.

- Heart attack

The heart attack occurs when there is a narrowing or complete occlusion of the coronaries, which bring oxygenated and nutrient-rich blood to the heart cells. A sudden interruption of blood flow leads in a few minutes to cell suffering and subsequently to the vascularized tissue's death from these arteries.

- Kidney failure

Kidney failure is the medical term that indicates an inability by the kidneys to properly perform its functions (clean up the blood from waste products, adjust the hydro-saline and acid-base balance of the blood, produce erythropoietin, etc.). Those suffering from kidney failure suffer from a serious health condition that deserves adequate and timely treatment.

- Lower limb amputation

This surgery practice is necessary when gangrene is developed in the lower limbs. It can be eaten or less depending on the size of the gangrene. When the ability to feel the toes is lost, they can frequently be injured without the person noticing, and, often, an ulcer can develop from a wound and can become a serious infection. Foot infections can spread all the way to the leg.

- Blindness

Most eye diseases associated with diabetes begin with blood vessel problems. Damaged blood vessels can cause damage to the retina and cause diabetic retinopathy.

Treatments

Before starting any treatment for insulin resistance, please contact your doctor. He will recommend the most suitable method for each person based on the cause that triggered it. While this guide will only offer useful advice. There are several effective ways to reduce the effects of insulin resistance from following proper nutrition to drug treatments. Of course, what can have a very strong impact on improving metabolic syndrome is a lifestyle change. Now let's see in detail all the possible treatments:

- Healthy nutrition

Regulating nutrition is the basis for a healthy life in general. For those suffering from insulin resistance, nutrition is the first cause of the onset of the pathology. Very often, those suffering from insulin resistance are overweight or obese. Thus, losing weight is a fundamental step that a person must take to avoid or treat this ailment and all its complications. To lose weight in an insulin resistance condition, the goal is always to maintain the optimal blood glucose level. In doing so, insulin is produced correctly, acting both on the metabolism of proteins and fats. To do this, eat small and frequent meals every day (5-6) to keep your blood sugar under control, always paying attention to the glycemic index of the foods you choose. In this sense, the most important meal is breakfast, which you should never skip not to worsen the condition of insulin resistance. In the next chapter, we will go into more detail on what to eat and avoid.

- Physical activity

The treatment of insulin resistance involves a 360 ° involvement of one's lifestyle, which cannot fail to include regular physical activity. Sport is the only factor that improves insulin sensitivity. Even regardless of the diet! Exercising regularly can help prevent diabetes by lowering the percentage of blood sugar and reducing body fat and overall weight. In fact, you have to remember that muscle is the place of greatest glucose consumption. Inactive muscle is not so sensitive to insulin action: that's why the movement is an essential factor in counteracting insulin resistance. It is therefore recommended to practice at least 2.5 / 3 hours of physical activity weekly. Many doctors recommend doing sports for 30/60 minutes every day, choosing moderate-intensity exercise: brisk walking is an excellent activity. Swimming, dancing, running are excellent sporting choices. However, it is unnecessary to practice strenuous sports: anything that keeps the body moving, and therefore also walking, is beneficial for the body. Also, opt for more dynamic choices in everyday life, such as using the stairs instead of the elevator or taking a walk during lunch break or parking far from the destination and then reaching it on foot.

- Drug therapy

Drug therapy is reserved only for those cases in which the change in lifestyle is not sufficient. In the case of insulin resistance diagnosed, it is advisable to contact your doctor to develop a targeted therapeutic plan and monitor its effectiveness. Drug therapy is aimed at decreasing the blood sugar level. The drugs that are used are oral hypoglycaemics, the most used to counter insulin resistance, we find:

- **Biguanidi**: indicated mainly for insulin resistance from obesity, as it has the effect of reducing hunger loss.
- **Glinidi**: are drugs that are used after every meal and that are used to lower blood sugar.
- **Sulphonylureas**: they act by increasing the sensitivity of cells to insulin and are the ones with the greatest efficacy. They are not always given because of their contraindications. They can alter plasma proteins.

- Natural remedies

Natural remedies are to be associated with adequate nutrition and are useful for lowering blood sugar levels. In this way, the insulin cell receptors will not be excessively stimulated, and the healing process can begin. We can make use of fennel herbal teas, nettle leaves, blueberry leaves, walnut leaves, and sage leaves among the natural preparations.

Diagnosis and exams

The diagnosis of insulin resistance is mainly based on evaluating the blood glucose and insulinemia values in the fasting patient. To diagnose insulin resistance with precision, sophisticated techniques performed in the laboratory are therefore necessary.

The most used are:
- **Blood glucose measurement**: usually done on an empty stomach. A glucose tolerance test may also be performed in some situations, with repeated measurements after a glucose load.
- **Glycated hemoglobin**: This test allows you to estimate increases in the average glucose concentration in the 3 months before the test. It is carried out by measuring the percentage of glycated hemoglobin present in the blood.
- **Lipid profile**: includes the complete measurement of triglycerides, total cholesterol, the good and bad cholesterol.
- **HOMA index**: this is a test that calculates insulin sensitivity by comparing plasma glucose concentrations and fasting insulinemia based on a mathematical model. In this way, the evolution of a possible metabolic syndrome can be assessed.

Chapter 2: Insulin resistance prevention

It is impossible to influence some risk factors for type 2 diabetes, such as insulin resistance and genetics. However, a person can take some measures to reduce the chances of insulin resistance. Some of the same strategies are critical for preventing heart disease and stroke. In addition, scientific studies report that individuals can reduce the risk of type 2 diabetes by changing their preventative lifestyle, primarily by losing weight and increasing physical activity. Muscles become more sensitive to insulin after exercise, and a person can reverse insulin resistance with an active and healthy lifestyle. Lifestyle changes have been shown to reduce the risk of progression to diabetes by more than 58 percent. Gradually increase your physical activity levels, replace one meal per meal with a healthy low-carb option, and make sure you keep it week by week. The most effective way to reduce insulin resistance is to make slow and sustainable changes. To prevent insulin resistance, therefore, it is necessary to take care of your lifestyle. This means eating in a healthy and balanced way and playing sports with consistency and regularity. Weight loss is also the best way to prevent blood glucose levels from getting too high. You must not forget that you can reverse this situation through healthy lifestyle choices, even if you have been diagnosed with an insulin resistance condition.

How can food help?

It is essential to know what to eat with insulin resistance. Regulating nutrition is one of the fundamental steps to prevent insulin resistance. Incorrect nutrition is the first cause of insulin resistance to arise in which people are often overweight or obese. Therefore, the migration and the correct choice of food is a crucial step for your well-being. Now let's see specifically the foods to eat and those to avoid.

What to eat
Here is a list of foods that make up a good diet for insulin resistance, so as not to excessively raise blood glucose levels:

- **Vegetables** - Vegetables are low in calories and rich in fiber: for this reason, they are the ideal food for people who try to manage the level of insulin in the blood. The best options are fresh vegetables such as tomatoes, spinach, peppers, cabbage, broccoli, cauliflower, and Brussels sprouts. On the other hand, although they may seem a healthy option, vegetable centrifugates do not satiate like non-centrifuged vegetables and contain much less fiber, eliminated in the centrifugation process.

- **Fruit** - Opt for fruit that contains much dietary fiber such as apples, berries, pears, plums, and peaches. Also, in this case, it is better to avoid the juices because they contain a lot of sugars and can, therefore, raise the blood glucose level.

- **Dairy products** - Dairy products contain calcium, which helps make teeth and bones stronger. Opt for partially or completely skimmed milk and yogurt with no added sugar. Whole milk and yogurt with added sugars are rich in saturated fats, the consumption of which in turn leads to insulin resistance. If you are lactose intolerant, you can try vegetable alternatives based on rice, soy, almonds, and rice.

- **Whole grains** - Whole grains are rich in vitamins, fiber, and minerals and perfect for insulin resistance patients. Some people think that avoiding carbohydrates is important for preventing diabetes, but in reality, whole grain and unprocessed carbohydrates are a good source of energy for the body. It is important to choose whole and unprocessed cereals and combine them with other healthy foods during meals, such as unsaturated fats and vegetables. Examples of "healthy" cereals are bulgur, oat flakes, brown corn, and brown rice, oats, and quinoa.

- **Beans and legumes** - Beans are an excellent source of fiber and therefore raise blood glucose levels very slowly. Some healthy options are borlotti beans, Lima beans, and black beans.

- **Fish** - Fish is rich in Omega-3 and good fats that help lower the risk of heart disease, very common in people who have diabetes. Omega-3 rich fish includes salmon, mackerel, herring, sardines, and trout. Cod and plaice are also healthy options but contain less Omega-3 because they contain less fat. Seafood lovers can consume lobsters, scampi, oysters, and mollusks, but they are cholesterol-rich foods. It is better to avoid breading and fries of these fish or if you choose to opt for fried fish, which is at least cooked with olive oil.

- **Chicken** - To consume a healthy variant of chicken, it is good to consume it without skin, which, in fact, contains more fat than the meat itself.

- **Lean proteins** - Among the proteins of animal origin, the fillet or ribs of pork or angel are especially recommended. Among vegetable proteins are a very valid option soy, tempeh, beans, and legumes: they are, in fact, excellent food choices.

- **Unsaturated Fats** - Unsaturated fats slow down digestion and are contained in dried fruit and seeds, low in carbohydrates. However, it is good to check the dried fruit packets' preparation because, in some cases, they contain a lot of sodium or added sugars, which increase calories and decrease their nutritional value. Avocado and olives could also be an optimal choice.

What to avoid

List of foods to avoid:

- **Fatty meats:** offal, seasoned meats, hot dogs, hamburgers, sausages, bacon. Red meat not prohibited but eat in moderation, no more than once a week.
- **Dairy products:** whole milk, cream, fatty cheeses, and whole yogurt.
- **Sweetened drinks:** Alcohol, carbonated drinks, fruit juices, and bottled tea.
- **Sweets:** candies, creams, chocolate, nougat, croissants, cakes, brioches, biscuits, sugar, and brown sugar.
- **Sauces and condiments**: mayonnaise, ketchup, creams, cake sauces, etc.

- **Fruit**: bananas, grapes, figs, tangerines, canned or candied fruit
- **Fish:** canned or salted fish. To limit the bluefish.
- **Starchy foods:** refined cereals such as pasta, bread, biscuits, and rice.
- **Salt**: salt should be used in moderation as it can raise blood pressure
- **Potatoes:** potatoes are rich in starch and therefore, should be limited. It is advisable to boil them before consumption to eliminate part of the starch inside them.
- **Animal seasonings**: butter, cream, bechamel, lard.

Physical activity

In basic prevention and treatment, together with food, exercise will have a great impact on overall results. Exercise and good physical activity can help your body avoid many complications. Exercise activates all your organs, tissues and muscles. It also allows you to consume all or most of the energy consumed by food. Exercise, especially if aerobic, is an integral part of the prevention of insulin resistance.

Which sport to choose?

The organization of a typical training session generally includes:

- A HEATING PHASE: 5-10 minutes of low-intensity aerobic activity to prepare the heart, skeletal muscle, and lungs for a progressive exercise increase. Then another 5-10 minutes of gentle muscle stretching.

- A CENTRAL PHASE CHARACTERIZED BY THE PLANNED PHYSICAL ACTIVITY
- FATIGUE AT THE END OF THE SESSION: 5-10 minutes to gradually bring the heart rate back to basal levels.

Here is a shortlist of recommended and non-recommended sports:

RECOMMENDED SPORTS: Fast running, light running, swimming, skiing, tennis
AUTHORIZED SPORTS: Basketball, volleyball, soccer, dance, cycling, athletics, canoeing, rowing, artistic gymnastics.
SPORTS NOT RECOMMENDED: Combat sports, motorsport, underwater sports

Benefits of regular physical activity
A physical exercise done 3-4 times a week for at least 30-60 minutes leads to the general improvement of the metabolic control parameters:

- Increased insulin sensitivity
- Cardiovascular disease prevention
- Induces a less atherogenic lipid profile
- Reduces triglyceride levels
- Increases good cholesterol
- Reduces bad cholesterol
- Lowers blood pressure levels significantly in patients with hyperinsulinemia
- Promotes weight loss
- Increased blood flow to insulin-sensitive tissues
- Higher proportion of type I muscle fibers that are more sensitive to insulin action than type II fibers
- Reduction of total fat and in particular of "insulin resistant" abdominal fat

Lifestyle

Insulin resistance can be prevented with a healthy lifestyle. By correcting nutrition and habits, much can be done to prevent this disease. Let's see how. Some environmental factors and lifestyles can favor the onset of insulin resistance. By correcting some bad habits, it is possible to do a lot to prevent diabetes and to cure it when the disease has already appeared. Let's see below how to fight diabetes with the correct lifestyle.

Eat healthy

The first thing you need to do is to eat healthy food. If you are eating elaborate meals, refined sugar, and other things, replace them with healthier alternatives. These unhealthy foods must be consumed on rare occasions. It is necessary to make food options healthy to avoid such problems and complications.

Organize your meals

Make sure you eat your meals on time at specific intervals. Eating large meals or eating long breaks can never be healthy. You need to feed your body with a small meal after a specific interval. Eating little and often will help you not eat large meals and will not make you hungry with the risk of bingeing.

Manage your stress

Stress and anxiety are not ideal for a healthy life if you continue to stress your body. Make sure to keep the right balance between working life and free time to relax and avoid health complications. A stressful brain affects the general functions of the body.

Maintain a balance between food options

Lifestyle changes are not about abandoning all food options and limiting to a specific type of diet. It's about knowing how to balance your food options. We simply need to prioritize foods over others. You have to keep the balance between the food options you want and those you can have.

Do not sleep immediately after meals

It is not an ideal habit to sleep or lie down immediately after eating. Under such conditions, the stomach can't digest food properly.

Increase activity

Physical activity must be an integral part of your life. If you do not have good physical activity in your daily routine, you will make the muscles inactive, and consequently less sensitive to insulin.

Stop smoking

Cigarettes increased blood glucose values. Consider that cigarette manufacturers have always added sugar to tobacco to make it harder and easier to inhale. Smoking increases 44% of type 2 diabetes compared to non-smokers. So stop smoking for all the other well-known complications that smoking involves!

Chapter 3: Breakfast

1) Zucchini and onion omelette

Ingredients:
- **3 eggs**
- **Parmesan cheese 2 tbsp**
- **Zucchini 1**
- **Onion 1**
- **1 tablespoon olive oil**
- **Garlic 1**
- **Salt and Pepper To Taste**

Preheat the oven to 180 ° C. In a bowl, beat the eggs and the grated Parmesan together. Finely slice the onions and courgettes, and place them in a non-stick pan with the oil, salt, pepper and crushed garlic. Cook until softened. Remove the garlic and distribute the vegetables on the pan and pour over the egg and parmesan mix. Cook for 3 minutes so that the bottom of the omelette solidifies. Place the omelette in the oven and cook for 12 minutes or until the eggs compact. Loosen the edges of the omelette and turn it over onto a plate. Cut the omelette into 4 slices and serve hot.

2) Spring frittata

Ingredients:

- **Eggs 4**
- **Red peppers 300 g**
- **Yellow peppers 300 g**
- **Carrots 1**
- **Asparagus 200 g**
- **Leeks 100 g**
- **Garlic 1 clove**
- **Thyme 3 sprigs**
- **Marjoram 2 sprigs**
- **Wild fennel 2 sprigs**
- **Salt to taste**
- **Black pepper to taste**
- **Extra virgin olive oil 40 g**

Start washing all the vegetables under plenty of fresh running water. Scrape the asparagus stalks with a vegetable peeler to remove the hardest external parts, then cut the stalk into cubes and the tips in half. Finely chop the leek, then peel the carrots and also cut them into cubes. Continue with the peppers' cleaning: remove the upper part, then remove the white filaments and seeds inside them with a knife, then cut them into cubes. Place a non-stick pan with the oil and the garlic clove on the fire. When the garlic is golden brown, remove it from the heat and pour the carrots and leek, cook for 2 minutes, and season with salt and pepper. Add the yellow and red peppers, asparagus, and cook for another 10-12 minutes by pouring a ladle of water and stirring. In a separate bowl, beat the eggs and add the salt and pepper. Also, add the aromatic herbs: thyme, marjoram, and fennel. Stir with the whisk to mix all the ingredients. Once the vegetables are ready, turn off and add them to the beaten egg, mixing well with a teaspoon. Pour everything in a non-stick pan and cook covering with a lid for 6-7 minutes over medium heat. With the lid's help, turn the frittata over to cook it on the other side for about 3 minutes. Once ready, turn off and serve your spring frittata.

3)   Almond and apricot biscuits

Ingredients:
- **90 g wholemeal flour 95 g type 0 flour**
- **55 g brown sugar**
- **5 g of baking powder**
- **2 lightly beaten eggs**
- **2 tablespoons of skim milk**
- **2 tablespoons of canola oil**
- **2 spoons of dark honey**
- **half a teaspoon of almond extract**
- **155 g of chopped dried apricots**
- **60 g of coarsely chopped almonds**

Preheat the oven to 175 C. In a large bowl, combine the flour, brown sugar, and baking powder. Mix the mixture. Add the eggs, milk, canola oil, honey, and almond extract. Stir until the dough starts to be compact. Add the apricots and chopped almonds. With floured hands, mix until the dough is well blended. Put the dough on a long sheet of transparent film, with your hands try to give a flattened shape 30 cm long, 7 cm wide, and about 2 cm high. Lift the cling film and place the dough on a non-stick pan. Bake until golden brown, 25 to 30 minutes. Transfer everything to a sheet of parchment paper and allow to cool for 10 minutes. Leave the oven at 175 degrees. Place the cooled mixture on a cutting board. With a serrated knife, cut the diagonal across 24 slices 1.5 centimeters wide. Arrange the slices on the baking sheet. Return to the oven and cook until golden brown for 15 to 20 minutes. Transfer to a rack and let cool completely. Transfer to an airtight container for storage.

4) Carrot bread

Ingredients:
- **60 g of type 0 flour**
- **120 g of whole wheat flour**
- **5 g of baking powder**
- **cinnamon powder**
- **half a teaspoon of ground cinnamon**
- **a pinch of ground ginger**
- **75 g fat-free margarine at room temperature**
- **55 g brown sugar plus 2 tbsp**
- **80 ml of skim milk**
- **2 tablespoons of unsweetened orange juice**
- **2 beaten egg whites**
- **5 ml of vanilla extract**
- **5 g of grated orange zest**
- **170 g of finely chopped carrots**
- **15 g of finely chopped walnuts**

Heat the oven to 190 degrees, grease the 250 g bread mold with margarine. In a small bowl, combine the first 6 dry ingredients. To put aside. Using a mixer, or stirring vigorously by hand, mix the margarine cream and sugar in a large bowl. Beat the milk, orange juice, eggs, vanilla, and orange zest. Add and mix the carrots and walnuts. Add the other dry ingredients. Mix well. Put the batter into the mold. Bake for 45 minutes, check the cooking with a toothpick (it must be dry). Leave to cool in the mold for 10 minutes. Remove from the mold and allow to cool completely on a wire rack.

5)   Chocolate cookies

Ingredients:
- **100 g Lupine flour**
- **100 g 85% dark chocolate**
- **100 g Hazelnut milk**
- **2 tbsp water**
- **1 pinch Bicarbonate**

Put the dark chocolate on a plate, then melt it in the microwave or a water bath. Meanwhile in a bowl put the lupine flour, add the vegetable milk, 1 pinch teaspoon of baking soda and mix with a spatula to create a creamy mixture, add the melted chocolate and mix initially always with the spatula then with your hands wet with water cold, until a stick is created. Take about 20 grams of dough at a time, and with wet hands, create many cookies in the shape of well-rounded marbles. Arrange them gradually on a mold covered with parchment paper. Bake in the preheated oven at 180 degrees for 10 minutes. Open the oven and lightly squeeze each marble with a fork or spatula. Raise the oven to 220 degrees and continue cooking for another 2-3 minutes. Remove from the mold of the biscuits and let them cool. So once cooled, arrange them on a serving plate and serve for breakfast!

6)   Coconut milk

Ingredients:
- **200 g of grated coconut**
- **1L of water**

Soak the coconut in the boiling water, turn off the stove, and cover with a lid. Leave to infuse for 6 hours. After the recommended time, blend with a blender. Pass all the mixture obtained in a fine pass transfer what is left in the pass in a sachet for food, close it with a knot then make many holes with a needle. At this point, start to squeeze it to recover the milk left in the coconut pulp. When you are finished, transfer the milk to a tight, tall, hermetically sealed container. So put it in the fridge overnight. The next day goes to take the container back in the refrigerator, take all the fat layer on the surface, the remaining liquid is pure, healthy, and degreased coconut milk. You can use it for breakfast or make sweets such as creams, ice cream, cakes.

7) Breakfast cake

Ingredients:
- **4 eggs**
- **100 g Rye flour**
- **100 g Buckwheat flour**
- **130 g coconut sugar**
- **50 g Bitter cocoa powder**
- **100 g 85% dark chocolate**
- **35 ml flax seed oil**
- **10 g Cremor tartar**
- **1 pinch of salt**

Beat the egg whites with an electric whisk, whisk egg yolks, coconut sugar, salt with an electric whisk. Add cocoa, grated chocolate, a few flours at a time, cream of tartar, and oil. Turn off the whips. Add the whipped egg whites and mix with a spatula from the bottom up. Transfer the mixture to an oiled cake pan (or lined with parchment paper). Bake in the preheated static oven at 190 ° for about 25 - 30 minutes.

8)   Soft briquettes without sugar

Ingredients:

- **500 g soft wheat**
- **100 g Sukrin**
- **2 eggs**
- **5 g Fresh brewer's yeast**
- **15 g Dehydrated sourdough**
- **270 g Lactose-free milk**
- **60 g light butter**
- **1 vanilla bean**
- **To brush**
- **1 eggs**
- **2 tablespoons Lactose-free milk**

Put the milk, sukrin, oil and brewer's yeast in a container and blend with an electric blender for 2 minutes. Add eggs, sow vanilla and mix for another 4 minutes. As you work, add the flour sifted together with the dehydrated sourdough bit by bit. When the dough is well blended, transfer it to a floured work surface. Work it to create a smooth dough. Place it in a large bowl, cover with a cloth and let it rest for 3/4 hours. After the leavening time, turn the bowl upside down on the work surface and divide the dough into 10 pieces of 90 gr each. Then work each piece and give the oval shape, gradually placing them in a baking tray covered with parchment paper. Leave to rise for another 2 hours covered with a cloth to cover. At the end of the 2 hours, they must be tripled in volume. Remove the brioches and immediately turn on the oven at 170 degrees. Brush on each brioche with 1 beaten egg yolk and 2 tablespoons of milk. Bake in the static oven at

170 C for about 10 minutes, after this time check from the glass of the oven, if the surface of the sponges is colored, cover them with a sheet of silver paper and continue cooking for another 5 minutes, if it is not colored do not cover them and continue cooking for another 5 minutes. Take the brioches, and they are ready to be eaten hot or cold!

9)   Ricotta biscuits

Ingredients:
- **140 g soft wheat flour**
- **1/2 sachet Baking powder**
- **12 g Stevia**
- **110 g Light ricotta**
- **25 g olive oil**
- **40 g Milk**
- **to garnish**
- **50 g 85% dark chocolate**

Put in a bowl: flour, yeast, stevia, ricotta, oil, and milk. Mix first with a spoon then finish the dough with your hands. Place it between two oiled parchment paper sheets, then roll it out with a rolling pin in a generous 1 cm thick sheet. Cut out with a cookie cutter of your choice. Arrange the biscuits gradually on a baking tray covered with parchment paper. Bake in the preheated oven at 190 ° for 8 minutes. Meanwhile, melt the chocolate in the microwave or a water bath. Remove from the oven and dip one at a time in the melted chocolate.

10) Honey biscuits

Ingredients:
- **60 ml water**
- **50 ml olive oil**
- **40 ml Honey**
- **125 g wholemeal flour**
- **125 g Oat flour**
- **1 sachet of yeast**
- **Vanilla extract**
- **50 g 85% dark chocolate**

On the work, the surface put both flours. Make a dimple in the center where honey, oil, water (leave half a glass aside), vanilla extract, and finally, the instant yeast for biscuits dissolved in the half glass of slightly warm water. Stir first with a fork, then form a dough with your hands. Spread the dough between two sheets of oiled parchment paper, form a sheet of about 1 cm. Cut the biscuits using the appropriate molds (to taste). More or less 30 biscuits are obtained. Arrange the biscuits gradually in a baking tray covered with parchment paper. Bake in the preheated oven at 180 degrees for 10 minutes. In the meantime, melt the chocolate in the microwave (or in a water bath). Remove the biscuits from the oven, let them cool down and dip them one by one in the melted chocolate. Leave them to thicken then arrange them in a tray.

11) Chocolate pancakes

Ingredients:
- 150 g almond flour
- 200 g water
- 2 teaspoons oil
- a pinch of salt
- ½ sachet baking powder
- 2 tablespoons of 85% melted dark chocolate

To garnish
- 1 tbsp honey

Put the flour in a bowl, then while adding the water mix quickly with an electric blender. Add the salt, oil and baking powder. Continue to stir the mixture until a smooth batter is obtained. Put a pan on the high heat, grease with a few drops of oil. Pour ½ ladle of batter into the center of the hot pan. Quickly pour 1 teaspoon of chocolate into the center of the batter. Cover immediately with 1 tablespoon of batter and cook for a few seconds. Check by lifting an edge with a spatula. Then turn the pancake and cook 10 seconds Transfer the cooked pancakes to a serving dish. Garnish with honey that has been drained.

12) Chocolate chip muffins

Ingredients:

- **Light softened butter at room temperature 60 g**
- **Almond flour 130 g**
- **Coconut sugar 70 g**
- **Room temperature skimmed milk 70 ml**
- **2 eggs**
- **Dark chocolate chips 50 g**
- **Vanilla bean 1**
- **Satin bicarbonate 1 tsp**
- **Salt up to a pinch**
- **Baking powder for cakes 10 g**

Work with the electric whisk butter, sugar until obtaining a frothy and creamy mixture. Then cut a vanilla bean and scrape the seeds with a knife. Pour the latter into the bowl with butter and sugar. Operate the whisk again and add the eggs one at a time. Now sift the flour, baking powder, and baking soda directly into the bowl with the mixture. Also, add a pinch of salt and operate the whips again to incorporate the powders. You will notice that the dough will become more consistent, then dilute it with milk at room temperature poured flush. At this point, the mixture will be soft and compact.

Add the chocolate chips and mix with a spatula to incorporate them. Then transfer the mixture into a disposable bag; thus, you can do a cleaner job; otherwise, use a spoon as well. Place the paper cups in a muffin pan and fill them 2/3 full. Each muffin will have to weigh approximately 70 grams. Pour the remaining chocolate chips over the cupcakes and bake in a preheated oven at 180 ° for 18-20 minutes in static mode. At this point, your chocolate chip muffins are ready to be enjoyed.

13) Low glycemic index waffles

Ingredients:
- **Almond flour 280 g**
- **Fat-free butter 220 g**
- **Eggs 6**
- **Baking powder for cakes 2 g**
- **Coconut sugar 180 g**
- **Vanilla bean 1**
- **Salt up to 1 tsp**

TO SEAL
- **Fresh fruit to taste**
- **Grated coconut**

First, melt the butter in the microwave or a water bath and let it cool. In the meantime, break the eggs at room temperature in a bowl, beat them lightly with a whisk, and then add the sugar and mix again. Sift the flour and baking powder directly into the bowl, add the salt and mix, first and then more and more vigorously with the whisk to mix the powders to the mixture and remove any lumps. Once it has cooled, pour the melted butter into the bowl a little at a time, to gradually incorporate it with the whisk. Extract the seeds from the vanilla pod with the blade of a knife, then add them to the mixture and mix again until a fairly dense and homogeneous consistency is obtained. Cover the bowl with plastic wrap and let the dough rest in the refrigerator for at least an hour. After the rest time, take out the dough and heat the waffle iron. When the plate is hot, brush it with a little melted butter and pour a little ladle of dough into the mold. Close the plate and cook for about 7-8 minutes. Check halfway through cooking. When the waffles have taken on a beautiful golden color, open the lid, gently remove them from the plate and transfer them to a plate. Garnish your delicious waffles with fresh fruit and grated coconut.

14) Sandwich with raw ham, avocado and tapenade

Ingredients:
- **16 slices of whole wheat bread**
- **350 g of raw ham**
- **1 ripe but firm avocado**
- **100 g of light fat-free butter**
- **1 jar of tapenade**
- **1 small shallot**
- **1 lemon**
- **small leaves of lettuce hearts**
- **salt**

Let the butter soften. Finely chop the shallot. Peel, pitted the avocado, cut it into slices, sprinkle them with lemon juice and a pinch of salt. Coarsely chop the ham. In a bowl, mix the butter and shallot until creamy, spread a light film on the surface of 8 slices of bread, spread the other four on both sides. On four slices buttered on one side spread the avocado slices, overlap four other buttered on both sides. On this spread, the chopped ham lay lettuce on it. Overlap the remaining buttered slices on both sides, spread them with the tapenade, lay a lettuce leaf on them. Overlap the remaining slices on the buttered side. Press everything lightly. With a knife with a very sharp blade, cut the sandwiches diagonally. Arrange the triangles obtained on as many white or colored paper napkins so that guests can easily use them.

15) Apple pie

Ingredients:
- **Apples 500 g**
- **Coconut sugar 100 g**
- **Almond flour 125 g**
- **Fat free butter 50 g**
- **Skimmed milk 75 g**
- **Eggs (at room temperature) 1**
- **Lemons 1**
- **Baking powder 8 g**
- **Cinnamon powder ½ tsp**
- **Salt up to a pinch**

Melt the butter in the microwave or a water bath, and keep it aside. Grate the lemon zest and squeeze the juice, then keep both the zest and the juice aside. Take the apples and slice them. Put the sliced apples in a bowl and drizzle with the lemon juice, mixing them well. Then move on to sift the flour with the baking powder. Then, in a large bowl, pour the eggs and part of the sugar dose. Begin beating with the electric whisk and continue pouring the sugar little by little. When the mixture starts to lighten, add a pinch of salt and continue whipping until you get a light and frothy dough. At this point, add the melted butter. Season with the cinnamon powder and also add the grated lemon zest. Then, continuing to whip with the whisk, add the sifted flour and baking powder a spoonful at a time. When the powders are completely incorporated, lower the electric whisks' speed and pour the milk flush at room temperature. When the milk is completely incorporated, stop the whips: the dough is ready. Separately, drain the apples in a colander to remove the lemon juice and pour them into the dough. Gently mix from bottom to top to incorporate them well. Grease and sprinkle a 22 cm diameter cake tin with sugar and pour the mixture using a spatula. The cake is ready to be baked: bake it in a preheated oven at 180 ° for about 55 minutes. When cooked, let it cool before removing it from the pan and enjoy it!

Chapter 4: Appetizers and Snacks

1) Crusted eggs

Ingredients:
- **4 eggs**
- **Onion 1/2**
- **Sliced wholemeal bread g 100**
- **Extra virgin olive oil**
- **Salt (to taste) 2 tbsp**
- **Handful of grated cheese**

In a grill or plate, toast the bread well. Shelves. Fry the onion in a pan with a little oil. Meanwhile, in a bowl, add the eggs and beat them with a whisk. Adjust with a pinch of salt and pepper. When they are well whipped, pour in the pan with the onion. Cook slowly until the eggs become creamy. Once ready, pour them on the previously toasted bread, sprinkle everything with Parmesan cheese.

2) Stuffed mushrooms

Ingredients:
- **Mushrooms (large) g 500**
- **Mayonnaise (fat free) n.2 tbsp**
- **Balsamic vinegar n.2 spoons**
- **Breadcrumbs 5 tbsp**
- **Chives n.2 spoons**

Preheat the oven to 200 C. Clean, wash the mushrooms, and deprive them of their stem. Chop the stalks together with 3 tablespoons of breadcrumbs, mayonnaise, chives, and vinegar. Fill the mushroom chapels with the mixture obtained and place them in a lightly greased pan with oil. Sprinkle with the remaining breadcrumbs and bake at 200 degrees for about 30 minutes, until the tops are golden brown.

3)   Chickpea balls with sesame

Ingredients:
- **Dried chickpeas 200 g**
- **Garlic cloves 1**
- **Small onion 50g**
- **Fresh coriander to taste**
- **Juice of half a lemon**
- **Cumin powder 1 tbsp**
- **Sesame seeds to taste**
- **Extra virgin olive oil 20g**
- **Salt to taste**

Soak the chickpeas for at least 8 hours. Boil them in abundant lightly salted water and cook them until they become soft. Drain the chickpeas and put them in a container and blend them. Add finely chopped garlic, onion, and coriander and mix everything. Then add the cumin, turmeric, and lemon juice. Season with salt and mix until a uniform dough is obtained. Let it rest for about thirty minutes. Prepare round meatballs to sprinkle with sesame seeds. Prepare an oven dish with extra virgin olive oil. Arrange the meatballs and bake at 165-170 ° C. Serve the meatballs hot.

4)   Baked pepper rolls

Ingredients:
- **Yellow peppers 1**
- **Red peppers 1**
- **2 tbsp breadcrumbs**
- **Salted anchovies 1**
- **1 sprig chopped parsley**
- **Pickled capers 1 tsp**
- **Basil 3 leaves**
- **Salt to taste**
- **Black pepper to taste**
- **Garlic 1 clove**
- **Diced mozzarella 20 g**

To prepare the roasted pepper rolls, start by cleaning the peppers with a damp cloth and placing them whole and unhulled in a pan. Bake them in the oven at 250 ° for about 20-25 minutes, turning them on the sides until the skin is wrinkled and brown. In the meantime, dedicate yourself to the filling: chop the parsley and the desalted and diluted anchovy. Place the mozzarella on a cutting board and slice it into cubes. Then place the breadcrumbs in a large bowl and add the minced anchovy and capers. With the appropriate tool, chop the garlic directly into the mixture, salt, and pepper to taste and add the chopped parsley. Finally, chop the basil leaves with your hands and add them to the filling. When the peppers have cooled, remove the green peduncle and peel them: the skin will come off easily, but be careful not to break them during this operation. Open the peppers, remove the inner seeds, and make 8 fairly wide layers. Place the flaps well open on a cutting board, sprinkle them with the previously prepared breadcrumbs mixture. In the center of each stratum, then arrange a couple of small cubes of mozzarella. Gently roll the stuffed peppers into rolls and arrange them in an ovenproof dish, which you will have lightly oiled previously. Bake for about 10 minutes at 200 ° and then take out of the oven: your baked pepper rolls are ready to be served warm!

5)   Chunks of quinoa

Ingredients:
- **Quinoa 150 g**
- **Small zucchini 2**
- **Eggs 1**
- **Grated cheese 50 g**
- **Grated lemon zest 1**
- **Fresh ginger to be grated to taste**
- **Salt to taste**
- **Black pepper to taste**

Preheat the oven to 180C. To prepare the quinoa morsels, start by placing the quinoa in a bowl and rinsing it under cold water until the water is clear. Boil the quinoa in a non-stick pan with salted water for the minutes indicated on the package (about 15-20 minutes), until the beans have absorbed most cooking water, softening and swelling. Proceed by draining the quinoa and passing it under cold water to stop cooking. At this point, wash the zucchini carefully and clean them. Then peel and peel the fresh ginger too. Grate the zucchini and place them in a large bowl, where you will add the grated lemon zest and the grated fresh ginger. Add the boiled quinoa to the grated zucchini, the ginger and the lemon zest, also add the grated cheese and the egg. Add salt and pepper to taste and mix the ingredients until a homogeneous mixture is obtained. Proceed by placing the mignon paper cups (about 4-5 cm in diameter and about 3 cm high) on a baking sheet and fill them with the mixture; you can also use a non-stick mold for mini muffins. Keep in mind that each cup in the photo contains approximately 20 g. Compact the mixture inside the baking cups with the back of a spoon to better define the morsels' shape. You just have to bake them in a preheated oven at 180 ° for 25 minutes, until the surface reaches a pleasant browning. At this point, the quinoa morsels are ready to be served and served warm!

6) Millet meatballs

Ingredients:
- **Organic peeled millet 200 g**
- **Water 550 g**
- **Extra virgin olive oil 25 g**
- **Gluten-free breadcrumbs 50 g**
- **Parsley (to be minced) 5 g**
- **Turmeric powder 1 pinch**
- **Salt up to a pinch**
- **Garlic 1 clove**
- **Zucchini 100 g**
- **Carrots 100 g**
- **Shallot 15 g**
- **Aubergines 100 g**

FOR BREADING AND COOKING
- **Gluten-free breadcrumbs 40 g**
- **Extra virgin olive oil 20 g**

FOR THE CREAM OF BEANS
- **Broad beans (shelled) 150 g**
- **Mint 2 leaves**
- **Extra virgin olive oil 10 g**
- **Salt up to a pinch**

Rinse the millet well under a stream of cold water and drain it, finely chop the shallot, and dice the carrot. Cut the aubergine and zucchini into cubes and put everything aside. Then heat the oil in a pan and add the millet, let it toast for a few minutes, stirring occasionally, then pour in hot water, add the salt and cook for 25 minutes. Once cooked, transfer the millet into a bowl and let it cool completely. In another pan, cook the shallots in a drizzle of oil over low heat, add the carrots, then the aubergines, and finally the zucchini. Salt all, and cook for 20 minutes, blending with a ladle of hot water or vegetable broth until they become soft. Now dedicate yourself to the fava bean cream preparation: shell them one by one, and once you have shelled all of them, blanch them for about 10-15 minutes. Then pour the beans into a container with high edges, add oil, mint, and salt and blend everything with an immersion blender until you get a creamy mixture. Add to the cold millet: the vegetables, the chopped parsley, a crushed clove of garlic, and the turmeric. Finally, add 50 g of gluten-free breadcrumbs to obtain a consistency suitable for working the meatballs. Then model the meatballs by taking about 25 g of the mixture and giving around and slightly flattened shape, then passing each meatball in the breadcrumbs and continuing until you finish the dough. Cook the meatballs in a non-stick pan in a little extra virgin olive oil, making them brown well on both sides to obtain a crisp and tasty surface. Serve your millet meatballs with vegetables as an appetizer.

7) Gratin tomatoes

Ingredients:

- Chopped parsley 2 tbsp
- Garlic 1 clove
- Salt to taste
- Black pepper to taste
- Anchovies in oil 20 g
- Vegetable broth 80 ml
- Extra virgin olive oil 15 ml
- Gluten-free breadcrumbs 55 g
- Pickled capers 8 g
- Chopped basil 6 leaves
- 4 firm and ripe coppery tomatoes 600 g

Preheat the oven to 200C. To make the gratin tomatoes, get 4 firm copper tomatoes weighing about 150 gr each which are more or less regular to each other. Wash the tomatoes under running water, then cut the tomatoes to about ¾ of their height, keeping aside the cap with the stalk that will serve as a garnish for the final dish. With a small knife, dig the pulp all around the circumference of the tomato and then, with a teaspoon, extract it; salt the inside of the tomatoes and place them upside down on a wire rack to drain (for about 20 minutes), so that they lose the vegetation water. Put the breadcrumbs in a bowl, drain the anchovies from the conservation oil and mince them and add them to the breadcrumbs, also drain the pickled capers and add them to the filling, the crushed garlic, the chopped parsley and basil, the oil, salt and broth by pouring it a little at a time, until the filling is soft. Now take the tomatoes and stuff them with the filling with the help of a spoon, grease an oven dish with oil, lay the tomatoes inside and cook in a static preheated oven at 200 ° for about 40 minutes. As soon as the tomatoes are slightly wrinkled and the surface is golden brown, take them out of the oven, let them cool, transfer them to a serving dish and garnish them with the upper cap that you have set aside.

8) Veal with tuna sauce

Ingredients:
- **Veal walker 800 g**
- **Celery 1 rib**
- **Carrots 1**
- **Golden onions 1**
- **Garlic 1 clove**
- **White wine 250 g**
- **Water 1.5 l**
- **Bay leaf 1 leaf**
- **Cloves 3**
- **Extra virgin olive oil 3 tbsp**
- **½ teaspoon black pepper**
- **Salt up to 2 pinches**

For the sauce
- **Eggs 2**
- **Drained tuna in oil 100 g**
- **Anchovies in oil 3 fillets**
- **Capers in salt 5 g**

Wash, peel the carrot, peel it, and cut it into pieces. Then remove the ends from the celery and also cut into pieces.

Peel the onion and divide it into 2 parts. Gradually collect the ingredients in a bowl and also add the whole garlic without a shirt. Switch to cleaning the meat by removing any cartilage and fat filaments. In a large saucepan, put the piece of walker, the cut vegetables, the bay leaf, 2-3 cloves, and the black peppercorns. Pour in the white wine and then the water that will cover it all. Add two pinches of salt and then the oil. Turn on the stove and wait for it to boil, after which, gradually remove the foam that will surface. Then close with the lid and slightly lower the heat, leaving to cook for about 40-45 minutes: remembering that for every 500 g of meat, it takes about 30 minutes of cooking. The important thing is that the meat does not exceed 65 ° in the heart, to be measured with a kitchen thermometer. Once the piece of meat is cooked, drain it and let it cool completely. Then remove bay leaf, pepper, and cloves. Recover 1/3 of the broth obtained and let it shrink over high heat for about ten minutes. When cooked, drain the vegetables in a bowl. Meanwhile, go ahead and prepare the hard-boiled eggs. In a saucepan with plenty of cold water, dip the fresh eggs. Turn on the stove and from the moment of boiling count 9 minutes. When they are firm, drain and rinse them under cold water. Once cooled, shell them and cut them into 4 parts. Add the egg segments to the bowl with the vegetables. Also, add the drained tuna, the anchovies in oil, and the desalted capers, finally, add a little broth. Use the hand blender and add more broth as needed. Blend until you get a smooth cream and the consistency you prefer. At this point, the meat should be completely cold. Slice it thinly with a smooth blade knife. Arrange the slices on a serving plate and pour the cream into the middle. Finally, decorate with the caper fruits, some whole and some cut in half, and your veal with tuna is ready.

9)   Mediterranean eggplant rolls

Ingredients:
- **Long aubergines 4 slices**
- **Mozzarella 100 g**
- **Tomato sauce 200 g**
- **Pitted olives 15 g**
- **Basil 4 leaves**
- **Garlic 1 clove**
- **Extra virgin olive oil 2 tbsp**
- **Salt to taste**
- **Black pepper to taste**

First, start preparing the sauce: heat the oil in a saucepan, add a clove of garlic and cook it for 5 minutes over low heat. When the oil has been flavored, pour the tomato pulp, salt, pepper, and cook for 15 minutes. While the tomato sauce is cooking, wash the aubergine and cut it into slices about 1 cm thick with a mandolin's help: you will have to make 4 long slices of uniform thickness. Heat a plate well, grill the aubergine slices on both sides, and then transfer them to a plate or a cutting board. When the tomato sauce is ready, remove the garlic clove. Chop the mozzarella with your hands 8 and preheat the oven to 180 ° in static mode. Now you are ready to assemble the rolls: spread a layer of tomato on the aubergines' surface, add a little frayed mozzarella, a teaspoon of olives, and a basil leaf. Roll the eggplants so stuffed and place them in a small baking dish with the closure facing down. Finally, cover the rolls with a little tomato sauce and a few pieces of mozzarella. The rolls are now ready to be baked: cook them in the static oven preheated to 180 ° for about 10 minutes, just long enough to melt the cheese. Once baked, your Mediterranean eggplant rolls are ready to be savored again!

10) Sea Salad

Ingredients:
- **Clean mussels 1 kg**
- **Clams clean 750 g**
- **Shrimp clean 500 g**
- **Octopus clean 700 g**
- **Large squid clean 400 g**
- **Carrots 2**
- **2 ribs celery**
- **Laurel 4 leaves**
- **Parsley to taste**
- **Garlic 1 clove**
- **Pink peppercorns 2**
- **Black peppercorns 2**

TO CONDITION
- **Lemon juice 40 g**
- **Extra virgin olive oil 40 g**
- **Parsley to taste**
- **Salt to taste**
- **Black pepper to taste**

Cut the squid into rings and set aside. Cut the celery and

carrot into coarse chunks, put them together with the bay leaves, parsley and peppercorns in a pot full of water. As soon as this is boiling, immerse the octopus completely and cover with the lid, simmer for 30-35 minutes; from time to time, you can remove residues and foam from the cooking water. Before draining it, skewer the meat with the prongs of a fork to check the cooking: it must be softened but firm in the center. When it is ready, lift it, without throwing the cooking water, and put it in a colander to cool. The same cooking water as the octopus, boil the squid for 5-8 minutes, depending on the size, and then the prawns for 30 seconds. Drain and let cool. In the meantime, sauté a clove of garlic with a drizzle of oil in a non-stick pan. When the garlic is golden brown, pour the mussels and clams and cook covering with a lid, letting them open spontaneously: it will take about 5 minutes. After this time, check all the mussels and clams: those that have not opened will be thrown away. Turn off the heat and drain them. Empty the mussels and clams into a bowl, taking care to keep some of both for the final decoration of the dish. Transfer the cold octopus to a cutting board and cut the tentacles into small pieces measuring 0.5 cm. In a separate bowl, prepare the dressing: pour the lemon juice, the oil, salt, pepper, and chopped parsley, beat a few moments to emulsify with a fork or whisk and pour over the mixture. Stir, and your seafood salad is ready to be served!

11) Marinated anchovies

Ingredients:
- **Anchovies (anchovies) (chopped) 500 g**
- **Garlic 4 g**
- **Lemon juice 150 g**
- **Parsley 20 g**
- **Extra virgin olive oil 140 g**
- **Black pepper to taste**
- **White wine vinegar 20 g**
- **Salt to taste**

To prepare the marinated anchovies started by marinating: in a mixer pour the parsley together with a clove of garlic, and 40 g of olive oil and mince everything for a few moments. Squeeze the lemons, and collect the juice in a container together with the olive oil and season with salt and black pepper. Mix well with the help of a hand whisk or the prongs of a fork and, when the two compounds have joined together, add the chopped parsley. Continue to stir with the whisk, then keep the marinade aside. Meanwhile, move on to cleaning the anchovies; since these will not undergo any cooking, it is very important to ensure that these have been cut down during the purchase phase; for greater safety, it is recommended to freeze for at least 96 hours at -18 degrees (already gutted) and then thaw to use in the recipe. Remove the head, and remove the entrails and bones. Finally, rinse the fillets underwater, taking great care not to divide the fish into two halves. Place the cleaned anchovy fillets in a large container next to each other, pour the marinade you have prepared, and then cover with plastic wrap. Let stand for at least 5 hours at room temperature. After the necessary time, remove the cling film and pour the white wine vinegar, mix and finally, drain them slightly from the marinade and arrange the marinated anchovies on a serving plate to serve them and enjoy them as an appetizer!

12) Stuffed mozzarella

Ingredients:
- **Mozzarella 4**
- **Cherry tomatoes 80 g**
- **Basil a few leaves**
- **Dried oregano to taste**
- **Salt to taste**
- **Extra virgin olive oil to taste**

To make the stuffed mozzarella, first cut each mozzarella's shell to obtain a recess, cut the caps into cubes, and keep them aside. Place the mozzarella dug in a colander with the recess facing downwards to eliminate excess water. Wash and divide the tomatoes into quarters and pour them into a bowl where you will also add most of the mozzarella cubes, keep the rest aside, they will serve garnish. Season with olive oil, salt, pepper, dried oregano, finally scented with fresh basil leaves. Stir to flavor the mozzarella stuffed with this filling, lay some mozzarella cubes on the surface that you have kept aside, and serve your fresh and tasty stuffed mozzarella!Black pepper to taste

13) Fresh black bean salad

Ingredients:

- **Black beans 500 g**
- **Cherry tomatoes 150 g**
- **Basil 9 leaves**
- **Shallot 100 g**
- **Salt to taste**
- **Black pepper to taste**
- **Extra virgin olive oil 30 g**
- **Thyme 3 sprigs**

Preheat the oven to 200C. Place a large pot full of water on the fire and pour the beans as soon as it has reached the boil. Cook for about 35 minutes without the lid. In the meantime, clean the shallots and divide them into four parts. Wash the cherry tomatoes and cut them in half. Pour the cherry tomatoes and the shallots into a baking tray. Scented with fresh thyme leaves and then seasoned with 20 gr of olive oil. Stir to flavor and then cook in the central part of the preheated oven in static mode for 20 minutes at 200 °. When cooked, remove the pan from the oven and let it cool at room temperature. In the meantime, the 35 minutes of cooking the beans will have passed, add salt and continue cooking for another 5 minutes. Once finished, turn off the heat, drain the beans, transfer them to a bowl, and add the tomatoes and shallots cooked in the oven. Add salt, pepper, and season with 10 gr of olive oil. Stir to flavor and serve the bean salad on the plates, perfuming with fresh basil leaves.

14) Salmon roll

Ingredients:

- **Smoked salmon fillet heart 200 g**
- **Medium eggs 4**
- **Parmesan cheese to be grated 25 g**
- **Salt to taste**
- **Black pepper to taste**
- **Extra virgin olive oil 5 g**

FOR MUSHROOMS
- **Mixed mushrooms 150 g**
- **Extra virgin olive oil 15 g**
- **Garlic 1 clove**

FOR THE SPINACH
- **Fresh spinach 150 g**
- **Extra virgin olive oil 15 g**
- **Garlic 1 clove**

Preheat the oven to 180C. In a small bowl, beat the eggs with the whisk by hand or with a fork. Season with salt and pepper. Pour the cheese and keep on whipping to avoid lumps. Now take a 34x27 cm oven tray, then line it with parchment paper and brush it with oil. Pour in the mixture. Bake the omelette in a preheated static oven at 180 ° C for 15 minutes. While the omelette is cooking, dedicate yourself to the mushrooms: with a gentle rotating movement, remove the chapel from the stem and deprive them of the stem's final part. Then cut them into not too thick slices and finely chop the parsley. Sprinkle a non-stick pan with a drizzle of oil and brown the garlic. Add the mushrooms and parsley. Cook over low heat for 8-10 minutes, then season with salt and pepper. When they are cooked, remove the garlic and keep the mushrooms aside. Now take another non-stick pan and brown a clove of garlic with a drizzle of oil. Pour the spinach, cover the pan with the lid and let it dry for 5-6 minutes over low heat. When cooked, remove the garlic. Transfer the spinach to a colander placed on top of a bowl, letting the spinach release the excess water. Also, keep the spinach aside. Take the salmon and cut it in half, then into very thin slices lengthwise. At this point, the omelette will be ready: take it out of the oven. On a cutting board lay some cling film and transfer over the omelette by turning it upside down from the pan. Remove the parchment paper gently and leave to cool to room temperature. Taking care to leave 2 cm from each edge of the omelette, fill the center with the spinach. Above the spinach lay the mushrooms and the slices of salmon. Then begin to close the roll by gently lifting the edges and bringing it towards the center. The film should only facilitate the closing of the roll and not be closed inside the preparation. Roll up gradually until the whole omelette is wrapped. Then close the ends and place the omelette roll in the refrigerator to compact it for at least 1 hour. After the time, take it out of the refrigerator, remove the cling film, and cut it into slices. Your salmon roll is now ready to be enjoyed.

15) Shrimp tartare

Ingredients:
- **Shrimp 2 kg**

Cherry tomatoes 12

FOR THE SAUCE
- **Basil 20 leaves**
- **Mint 20 leaves**
- **Garlic 1 clove**
- **Extra virgin olive oil to taste**
- **Salt to taste**
- **Black pepper to taste**
- **Lemon zest 1**

To prepare the scampi tartare, make sure you have purchased slaughtered scampi, freeze them for 96 hours at -18 degrees for greater safety. Clean and shell the prawns and transfer the pulp to a cutting board. Lightly cut the central part of the pulp with a knife and remove the intestine. Divide the prawns in half and cut them into small cubes. Carry out the same procedure with all the prawns, then transfer them to a bowl, cover them well with plastic wrap and leave them in the refrigerator until used. At this point, wash the cherry tomatoes under running water and place them on a cutting board. Divide them, cut them into cubes, and keep them in a bowl until you are ready to use them. Now prepare the basil and mint sauce: quickly rinse the basil leaves and put them in the mixer, add the mint leaves, a peeled garlic clove, and the oil. Salt and pepper to taste and then whisk until a smooth and homogeneous sauce is obtained. At this point, take a serving dish and pour a spoonful of basil and mint sauce on the bottom, then place a 7 cm diameter pastry cutter in the center of the sauce and fill it halfway with the scampi, pressing well with a spoon, in so that the layer takes on the shape of the pastry cutter. Continue forming a layer of diced cherry tomatoes. Form another layer of diced prawns, press again, and leave in the fridge until ready to serve. Before bringing the scampi tartare to the table, remove the pastry cutter, garnish with the grated lemon zest and finish with a drizzle of oil: your scampi tartare is ready to be served and enjoyed!

Chapter 5: Meat

1) Escalope in white wine

Ingredients:
- Chicken breast slices 4
- Sage leaves 4
- Spoons of whole wheat flour 2
- Sprigs of rosemary 2
- Sage sprigs 2
- Bay leaf 1
- Garlic clove 1
- Glass of white wine 1
- Salt, pepper and extra virgin olive oil olive oil to taste

Take a pan and put it on medium heat with some olive oil. Take the chicken breasts and sprinkle the flour on each one, and put them in a pan. Add rosemary, sage, garlic clove, bay leaf, and brown everything together. Brown until both sides are slightly brown. Place the breasts on a plate without turning off the heat, drain the oil, and remove the perfumes. Put the chicken back in the same pan and cook with the white wine and add a little water. Season with salt and pepper. Cook until a sauce has been created, and the alcohol phase has evaporated. To serve.

2) Lamb chops with spring onions flavored with marjoram

Ingredients:

- **Lamb loin 400 g**
- **Red peppers 500 g**
- **Spring onions 500 g**
- **Extra virgin olive oil 40 g**
- **Vegetable broth 2 ladles**
- **Rosemary to taste**
- **Marjoram to taste**
- **Salt to taste**

Preheat the oven to 220 C. Remove the loin from the bone base and all the scraps to clean the piece of fillet. Brush the ribs with oil, salt, and bake at 220 ° for about 15 minutes, adding a rosemary sprig. Cut the pepper and spring onion into coarse pieces. Put them in a pan with oil and add salt and fresh marjoram. Add the vegetable stock and let it simmer. Serve the cut lamb chops, accompanied by the vegetable stew.

3) Rabbit stew

Ingredients:

- **Rabbit 350 g**
- **Seed oil 4 tbsp**
- **1 clove crushed garlic**
- **Chopped parsley g 10**
- **Dry white wine 3 tbsp**
- **Sliced tomato pulp 100 g**
- **Salt. g 15**

- **A pinch of pepper**

Heat the oil in a pan, add the rabbit pieces, sauté over medium heat, season with salt and pepper, the clove of garlic, and the chopped parsley. As soon as the garlic turns brown, remove it, pour the wine and let the alcohol evaporate. Add the tomato pulp and a few tablespoons of water. Continue cooking with the pan covered over low heat for twenty minutes. Serve with the thickened sauce.

4)   Chunks of chicken in fennel sauce

Ingredients:
- **Chicken breasts g 600**
- **Fennel n 3 medium**
- **Garlic cloves 2**
- **Dry oregano 1/2 tsp**
- **Chili powder 1/4 tsp**
- **Chopped onion 4 tbsp**
- **Extra virgin olive oil**
- **Salt and pepper**

In a large skillet, heat the oil and quickly brown the diced chicken over high heat. Brown on all sides, then drain and keep warm. In the same pan, add the chopped onion, garlic, and cook over low heat for a few minutes. Add the cleaned, washed, and thinly sliced fennel. Wet with two water glasses, add the salt, chili pepper, and oregano, cover, and simmer for about 20 minutes or until the water has dried, and the fennel is almost reduced to cream. Bring the chicken back on the heat, stir, and cook for another 5 minutes. Turn off and serve hot.

5) Roast turkey stuffed with broccoli

Ingredients:
- **Turkey breast 700 g**
- **Broccoli tops 250 g**
- **1 egg white**
- **Garlic 1 clove**
- **1 pinch chili**
- **2 tablespoons olive oil**
- **Salt to taste**

Preheat the oven to 180C. In a pot filled with salted water, boil the broccoli until tender. Drain just ready. In a pan heat 1 tablespoon of oil and brown the minced garlic for a few minutes. Add the tops of boiled broccoli and the chili pepper. Cook for a few minutes, until they are well flavored. Turn off and let cool, then add the egg white and mix well. On the cutting board, roll out the turkey breast, cut a side pocket, and stuff with broccoli. Close with kitchen string, brush with the rest of the oil and inform at 180 ° for 40 minutes. Turn once. If necessary, moisten with a little broth. Remove from the oven and leave to rest for a few minutes, then slice and serve hot.

6)   Spicy chicken skewers

Ingredients:
- **Chicken breast 500 g**
- **Garlic 1 clove**
- **Salt to taste**
- **Black pepper to taste**
- **Spicy paprika 1 tbsp**
- **Cayenne pepper 1 tbsp**
- **Honey 30 g**
- **Sesame seeds 10 g**
- **Extra virgin olive oil 30 g**

Take the chicken breast and cut it first into strips and then into cubes of about 2 cm. Transfer them to a bowl and add the oil. Salt, pepper, and add the spices too: first the cayenne pepper and then the paprika. Finally, add the honey, the crushed garlic, and mix everything. At this point, cover with cling film and store in the refrigerator to marinate for at least 2 hours, preferably overnight. After this time, take the steel (or wooden) skewers and stack the meat pieces, leaving a space between the various cubes. Once all the skewers are formed and sprinkle them with sesame seeds. Wait 3-4 minutes, until they are well toasted and lightly caramelized. Then turn them over, finish cooking for another 2-3 minutes, and serve your spicy chicken skewers.

7)   Stuffed roast

Ingredients:
- **Pork loin a single slice 700 g**
- **Sliced raw ham 140 g**
- **Vegetable broth 300 ml**
- **Carrots 2**
- **2 ribs celery**
- **Red onions 1**
- **Thyme 1 sprig**
- **Marjoram 1 sprig**
- **1 sprig rosemary**
- **Sage 1 leaf**

Start with the vegetables that will be used to cook the roast. Peel and peel the carrots, then divide them in half. Wash the celery stalks and cut them into rather large pieces. Then peel the red onion too and reduce this to rather large pieces. Put the vegetables aside. Then take the meat, put it on a cutting board, cover it with a parchment paper sheet, and beat it with the meat tenderizer to make it thin and tender. Then remove the sheet of parchment paper and lay the slices of raw ham on the meat. Then start rolling the roast well, gently so as not to spill the filling until it is completely closed. Now proceed to tie the roast with the kitchen string. Insert a sprig of marjoram, one of thyme and one of rosemary between the string. Then take a large pan, pour plenty of olive oil until it covers the bottom, add the roast, also turn it on the other side to brown it. Pour the vegetables you previously cut into the pan, then salt and pepper to taste. Pour the vegetable stock and cook with the lid on low heat for an hour and a half, occasionally turning the roast. After the necessary time, uncover it and put out the fire. Remove the roast and let it cool; pour the cooking juices into the mixer and blend it to obtain a thick sauce that you will use as an accompaniment. So when it has cooled, take the roast and place it on a cutting board, slice it to your liking. Your stuffed roast will then be ready to be served hot or warm accompanied with the vegetable sauce!

8)   Duck breast with balsamic vinegar

Ingredients:
- **Duck breast (2 pieces)**
- **Golden onions 100 g**
- **Garlic 1 wedges**
- **2 sprigs rosemary**
- **Thyme 2 sprigs**
- **Balsamic vinegar 40 g**
- **Honey 10 g**
- **Water or vegetable broth 100 g**
- **Mixed salad 50 g**

Remove excess fat from the chest with a knife's help and proceed to make cuts first obliquely and then vertically. Repeat the same operation for the other breast, too, then salt and pepper on both sides. Place a pan on the heat and let it warm up, when it is hot lay the duck breasts on the side of the skin. After 3-4 minutes, turn them over and let them brown on the other side. At this point, add the peeled onion cut into wedges and the poached garlic. Add thyme, rosemary, and blend with balsamic vinegar.

Let it evaporate slightly and add the water (or if you prefer vegetable broth). Cook the duck breast for about ten minutes (it will have to remain pink inside) then transfer it to a cutting board keeping the cooking base aside, which you will pour into a colander. Strain the liquid by crushing the mixture with a spoon directly in the same pan where you will have cooked the duck breast.

9)   Baked lamb chops

Ingredients:
- **Lamb chops 800 g**
- **Thyme 2 sprigs**
- **Rosemary 3 sprigs**
- **Salt to taste**
- **Black peppercorns to taste**
- **2 cloves garlic**
- **Extra virgin olive oil 40 g**
- **Lemon zest 1**
- **Black pepper to taste**

Start cleaning the meat from excess fat, then make cuts between one rib and the other and, with the help of your fingers, push the meat down to free the bone as much as possible. Transfer the ribs to an ovenproof dish and season with 4 salt and pepper. Also, add 2 sprigs of rosemary, thyme, and peppercorns. Pour about 10 g of oil, add the freshly grated lemon zest, and sprinkle all the ribs. Also, add a clove of garlic divided in half, cover with plastic wrap, and leave to marinate for about 2 hours in the refrigerator. Place the ribs on a lightly greased baking dish. Wrap the bones with a strip of aluminum foil, completely cover them and not let them burn during cooking. Then bake in a preheated static oven at 200 ° for 50 minutes. Once cooked, take out of the oven and serve your lamb chops in the oven.

10) Chicken in Green Sauce

Ingredients:
- **Chicken breast 600 g**
- **Parsley 20 g**
- **Basil 15 leaves**
- **Capers 20 g**
- **Pitted green olives 20 g**
- **Extra virgin olive oil 3 tbsp**
- **White onions 1**
- **Carrots 1**
- **Laurel 4 leaves**
- **Black peppercorns 10**
- **Garlic 1 clove**
- **Salt to taste**
- **Lemon juice to taste**
- **Green salad (optional) to taste**

Start by peeling and peeling the onion and cutting a carrot in two. Place them in about 1.5 liters of water and add the bay leaves and peppercorns. Salt and bring to the boil. Lower the heat and put the chicken breasts to boil; they will have to cook for 15 to 20 minutes depending on the thickness of the meat, which must be completely white. In the meantime, dedicate yourself to preparing the sauce in a mixer chop the olives, capers, basil, garlic, and parsley. Add 3 tablespoons of oil, a splash of lemon juice and mix everything. Add salt if necessary and if the green sauce turns out to be too thick, add a little oil, a little lemon juice or a little water to taste. Then drain the chicken breasts, let them cool, and cut them into regular strips. Put some salad in a bowl, add the strips of chicken breasts and season them with the green sauce obtained.

11) Baked spare ribs

Ingredients:

- **Pork ribs 1 kg**
- **1 sprig rosemary**
- **2 cloves garlic**
- **Paprika 1 tsp**
- **Salt to taste**
- **Black pepper to taste**
- **Extra virgin olive oil 20 g**

Preheat the oven to 160 C. Cut them into wedges, peel the garlic leaving the whole wedges, and cut them into 2 parts. In a large bowl, put the ribs, garlic, rosemary, and paprika. Season also with salt and pepper and season with oil. Mix well with your hands. Transfer everything to a large pan, cover with aluminum foil and bake in a preheated static oven for about 3 hours at 160 °. After 3 hours, remove the aluminum foil and raise the oven temperature to 220 °. Let them cook again for 45 minutes. Serve the ribs in the oven hot!

12) Crusted chicken legs

Ingredients:
- **Chicken legs 4**
- **Whole wheat bread 200 g**
- **Chopped parsley 3 tbsp**
- **2 cloves minced garlic**
- **Lemon zest 1 tbsp**
- **Extra virgin olive oil 4 tbsp**
- **Ground black pepper 1 tsp**
- **Salt up to 1 tsp**

Grate the bread. Season the crumb obtained with the grated lemon zest, salt, parsley, pepper, minced garlic cloves, and oil. Then mix everything with your hands, creating a breading where the ingredients must be mixed well. Then take care of the thighs, peel them if necessary, brush them with olive oil, then pass the thighs in the breading, make sure that it adheres well on both sides, and help you with your fingers by exerting light pressure. Preheat the grill to maximum power. Lower over medium heat and cook the thighs 7/8 minutes per side until a dark and crispy crust is reached. Serve with a lemon wedge.

13) Turkey rolls stuffed with Champignon mushrooms

Ingredients:

- **Sliced turkey 4**
- **Champignon Mushrooms 400 g**
- **Smoked scamorza 200 g**
- **Vegetable broth 50 g**
- **Extra virgin olive oil 20 g**
- **Garlic 1 clove**
- **1 sprig chopped parsley**
- **Pepper 1 pinch**
- **Salt 1 pinch**

Clean the champignon mushrooms: remove the most earthy part of the stem, clean them with a dry or slightly moistened cloth, and then cut them into thin slices. You can keep 300 g aside as a side dish, while 100 g will stuff the rolls. Cut the scamorza cheese into thin slices. Then place each slice of meat between two sheets of parchment paper and beat it with a meat mallet to decrease its thickness then cut each slice in half. Put a few slices of scamorza and some mushrooms on the turkey. Roll the roll on itself and stop everything with a toothpick. Proceed in the same way with all the rolls until you finish the ingredients. In a large pan, brown a whole clove of garlic with the oil, then add the rolls and brown them by turning them over to promote homogeneous cooking. Pour the 300 g of mushrooms aside in a pan, season with salt and pepper, and add the vegetable stock. Cover with the lid and continue cooking for 15-20 minutes. Once cooked, turn off the heat and serve the turkey rolls stuffed with hot Champignon mushrooms!

14) Leg Of Lamb Baked

Ingredients:
- **Leg of lamb 1,5 kg**
- **Extra virgin olive oil 30 g**
- **Salt to taste**
- **Black pepper to taste**
- **Rosemary 3 sprigs**
- **Thyme 3 sprigs**

Preheat the oven to 180C. First, try to free the final part of the bone from the meat so that it will not tend to curl during cooking. Then eliminate the part of excess fat on the whole leg, until it is almost completely cleaned. At this point, salt, pepper, and massage the meat with your hands. Then transfer it to a lightly greased pan and sprinkle the entire surface with a drizzle of oil. Cover with rosemary and thyme sprigs. Bake at 180 degrees for 50 minutes, placing it on the oven's bottom shelf, turning the leg halfway through cooking. Once it is well browned and perfectly cooked on both sides, serve your leg of lamb still steaming!

15) Turkey burger

Ingredients:

- **Wholemeal hamburger buns 4**
- **Ground turkey 600 g**
- **Aubergines 480 g**
- **Auburn tomatoes 320 g**
- **Green salad 60 g**
- **Rosemary to taste**
- **Oregano to taste**
- **Thyme to taste**
- **Salt to taste**
- **Black pepper to taste**
- **Extra virgin olive oil 10 g**

Start by chopping the aromatic herbs: rosemary, oregano, and thyme. In a bowl, add the minced meat with the mince; season with salt and pepper. Knead all the ingredients by hand and let the mixture rest in the refrigerator for 15 minutes. Meanwhile, wash and tick the aubergine removing the ends. Slice it about half a centimeter thick and place it on a well-heated and lightly greased plate. After a few minutes of cooking, turn the aubergine discs so you will also cook them on the other side at the end of cooking, set aside. Browse your salad and rinse it thoroughly to get rid of soil residues, then transfer the lettuce onto a tray with paper towels and gently dab it to dry; in this way, you will not damage it. Finally, wash the tomato and slice it in half centimeter thick slices after having stripped it of the stalk. At this point, all your ingredients are ready. Take the minced meat from the fridge and place it inside an 11 cm circular pasta bowl that you will have placed on a parchment paper sheet. Then help yourself with the back of a spoon to level the surface to smooth and brush each hamburger with a little oil.

Place the meat medallions on the hot grill, and after 4 minutes of cooking, you can turn them with the help of a spatula to cook them on the other side for the same time. If you want a well-warmed and slightly toasted sandwich, cut the bread into two parts, then arrange the two parts on the still hot grill, letting go for a few minutes, until the base has become crispy.

As soon as your sandwiches are hot, switch to the composition: then on the sandwich base lay 3-4 lettuce leaves and 4 tomato disks, then 4 slices of aubergines and finally your meat medallion. Close with the other half of bread, and your turkey burgers are ready to be bitten still hot!

Chapter 6: Fish & Seafood

1)   Trout fillet with spinach

Ingredients:
- **Trout fillets 4**
- **Spinach 200 g**
- **Grated Parmesan 20 g**
- **Onion ½**
- **Salt, pepper, olive oil to taste**

Preheat the oven to 180 C. Chop the onion and put it in a pan over medium heat with a drizzle of oil. Add the spinach and brown them together with the onion, salt, and pepper. When the spinach has wilted, remove from the pan and mince. Grease the oven pan with olive oil and place the trout fillets. Cover the trout fillets with the spinach and sprinkle with the Parmesan. Bake at 180 degrees for 15 minutes and serve.

2)   Cuttlefish with peas

Ingredients:
- **Cuttlefish or large cuttlefish cut into strips kg 1**
- **Fine peas 500 g**
- **Jar of diced tomato 1**
- **Medium onion 1**
- **Garlic cloves 3**
- **Sprig of rosemary 1**
- **White wine ½ glass**

Chop the garlic, onion, and rosemary finely and put them in a pan with the oil and chili pepper and fry. Pour the white wine, evaporate the alcohol, and add the tomato, salt, and cook for 15 min. Separately, in a saucepan with a little water and a little salt, pour the peas that will be cooked in a few minutes. Remove the peas from the pan and set aside. In the same water, cook the cuttlefish for 2 minutes. Drain the cuttlefish and add them to the tomato. Add the peas and the chopped parsley; bring back to the boil and cook for another minute. Ready to be served!

3) Cod fillets with creole sauce

Ingredients:
- **Fish fillets 4**
- **Lemon juice 2 tbsp**
- **Light margarine 4 tbsp**
- **Chopped green peppers 60g cup**
- **120g tomatoes**
- **Flour 1 tsp**
- **Chopped onion 2 tbsp**
- **Salt and Pepper To Taste**

Preheat the oven to 200 °. In a bowl, mix lemon juice, finely chopped onion, and 2 tablespoons of melted margarine. Place the mixture on top of the fish. Sprinkle a baking dish with oil, lay the fish fillets on it, and bake in the oven. Cook until the fork easily penetrates the fish fillet, about 15 minutes. While the fish is cooking, in a pan over medium heat, prepare the Creole sauce by browning the tomatoes and green peppers in the remaining margarine. Let the vegetables dry and add the flour and mix to have a creamy sauce. Remove the cod from the oven and put it on a plate, sprinkling the mixture over the fillet.

4)   Sole flavored with basil and mint

Ingredients:
- **Fillets of sole 4**
- **Chopped fresh basil 2 tbsp**
- **Chopped fresh mint 1 tbsp**
- **Garlic 1 clove**
- **Extra virgin olive oil 50 g**
- **Salt and white pepper**

Wash the fish fillets and dry them well with kitchen paper towels. Put a non-stick pan on the fire that you have previously greased with extra virgin olive oil and cook over medium heat. As soon as the pan is hot, place the sole fillets on top. Add a little salt, freshly ground pepper, and the mince you have prepared with the basil, mint, and garlic. Cook 3 minutes per side or until the inside is completely white. Season them with a drizzle of raw oil and serve hot.

5)   Shrimp with dried tomatoes

Ingredients:
- **Shelled and cleaned shrimp 500 g**
- **Anchovies 6**
- **Dried tomatoes 6**
- **A handful of capers**
- **Tomatoes 4**
- **Garlic cloves 3**
- **Pitted olives 10**
- **Lemon 1**
- **Black pepper to taste**
- **Parsley to taste**
- **Basil to taste**

Heat olive oil over medium-high heat in a large pan. Add the prawns, peeled and cleaned, with half a teaspoon of salt and half of black pepper; cook for 5 minutes, occasionally turning the prawns. Put the prawns in a bowl and keep them warm. Pour the wine into the pan, mix, and let it evaporate. Cut the fresh and dried tomatoes, add the garlic and cook in a pan over medium heat until everything is softened (about 3 minutes). Take the lemon, cut the peel and chop it, add the shredded anchovies, two tablespoons of capers, parsley olives, and basil. Cook for 2 minutes, mixing everything. Return the prawns to the pan and mix. Serve immediately.

6) Mussels in broth

Ingredients:
- **Clean mussels 1 kg**
- **Olive oil to taste**
- **Chopped shallots 1**
- **Garlic cloves 2**
- **White wine to taste**
- **Vegetable broth 240ml**
- **Ground pepper to taste**
- **Fresh parsley to taste**

In a large and deep pan, pour olive oil and fry garlic and shallots until they soften (about 5 minutes). Add the wine and let it evaporate. When you no longer smell the alcohol, pour the broth and half a spoonful of pepper, bring to the boil. Leave to cook for 5 minutes. Take the previously cleaned mussels and add them to the pan, cover, and cook until the mussels are completely open by shaking the pan often. Discard any mussel that has not opened. Divide the mussel broth into soup plates and sprinkle with 2 tablespoons of chopped fresh parsley.

7)   Risotto with seafood

Ingredients:

- **Brown rice 320 g**
- **Mussels 1 kg**
- **Clams 500 g**
- **Squid already cleaned 350 g**
- **Prawns (the tails) 300 g**
- **Parsley 1 sprig**
- **2 cloves garlic**
- **White wine 90 ml**
- **Vegetable broth to taste**
- **Extra virgin olive oil to taste**
- **Light cold butter 70 g**
- **Fresh spring onion 50 g**
- **Celery 25 g**
- **Carrots 25 g**
- **Chili pepper 1**
- **Salt to taste**
- **Black pepper to taste**

To prepare the risotto with seafood, start by cleaning all the mollusks and crustaceans. Start by cooking the mussels, put a large pot on the stove, turn on the maximum power, and pour them. Close with the lid and let them open by shaking the pot occasionally. It will take 2-3 minutes to open. Filter the liquid by pouring it into a colander placed in a container. Wait a few minutes before you start shelling them so that you won't get burned. Set aside 2-3 whole mussels for each plate, they will serve you for the final decoration. Switch to cooking the clams. Put the pan back on the stove, turn on the stove, and pour it inside. Close with the lid and leave them open by shaking the pot occasionally. The clams will hatch in 1-2 minutes, as soon as they are opened, filter the liquid by pouring it into the same container used to collect the mussel. Let cool a few moments before shelling these too, still holding 2-3 whole pieces for the plate.

Heat the vegetable broth and move on to cleaning celery, carrot and spring onion. Chop them finely with a knife; clean the garlic cloves leaving them whole. Finally, also clean the chili and then chop it, and chop the parsley. Put everything aside and move back to the stove. Put a saucepan on the fire, make a turn of oil inside and pour the chopped celery, carrots, spring onion, garlic, and chopped red pepper. Let everything flavor for about ten minutes on low heat, stirring occasionally. Once the odors have dried, eliminate the garlic, raise to a maximum temperature, and add the squid cut into pieces. Sauté them for 1 minute before adding the shrimp tails too. Blanch for another minute and, as soon as the liquid dries, blend with half the white wine. When the alcohol has completely evaporated, turn off and transfer the squid and prawns to a bowl, cover with the lid and leave warm. Pour the rice into the same pan and let it toast for about 1 minute at maximum power, constantly stirring, thus avoiding the beans burning. When they are toasted, blend with the remaining part of white wine and wait for the alcohol to evaporate before cooking the rice with the broth. You can wet it a little at a time with ladles until cooking is complete. Add the liquid of mussels and clams and mix occasionally, but not too much. When 1-2 minutes are left from the end of cooking, add the prawns

and squid, mussels, and clams and season everything.
Turn off and stir, adding the very cold and diced butter,
chopped parsley, and freshly ground black pepper. Stir
and let rest a few minutes before serving. Your seafood
risotto is ready garnished with mussels and clams kept
aside.

8)   Baked sea bream

Ingredients:
- **Sea bream 2 cleaned**
- **Garlic 1 clove**
- **Salt to taste**
- **Black pepper to taste**
- **Parsley 2 tufts**
- **Thyme 2 sprigs**
- **Extra virgin olive oil 20 g**
- **Lemons 1 slice**

Preheat the oven to 180C. Wash and chop the parsley.
Place a parchment paper sheet on a baking tray and place
each clean sea bream in the center, salt, and pepper the
inside. Then stuffed with the aromas: sprigs of thyme
previously washed and dried, half a clove of peeled garlic
for each sea bream, half a slice of lemon, and extra virgin
olive oil. Pour in a drizzle of olive oil also over the sea
bream, close the parchment paper sheet by rolling the
two ends. Then wrap it in aluminum foil, wrinkling the
ends in this case too to seal. Place the sea bream on a
baking sheet and bake in a preheated static oven at 180 °
for about 40 minutes. When cooked, take the sea bream
out of the oven, let it cool and then serve it in the same
foil, sprinkling it with fresh parsley if you like.

9) Spaghetti with tuna

Ingredients:

- **Whole wheat spaghetti 320 g**
- **Tuna in oil (drained) 150 g**
- **Peeled tomatoes 400 g**
- **Extra virgin olive oil to taste**
- **Salt to taste**
- **Black pepper to taste**
- **Basil to taste**
- **Golden onions ½**

To prepare the spaghetti with tuna, start by heating a pot full of water on the fire, salted when it is boiling: it will be used to cook the pasta. Drain the tuna fillet from the conservation oil. In the meantime, peel the onion, slice it thinly. Heat the olive oil in a pan and add the sliced onion. Let it dry on low heat for a few minutes, stirring often; fray the tuna with your hands and add it to the pan when the onion is softened and let it brown for a couple of minutes, stirring constantly. Now, mash the tomatoes with a fork and pour them into the pan with the tuna; let the sauce cook for about 10 minutes. Meanwhile, cook the spaghetti in the boiling water during the cooking time of the pasta. Cook the spaghetti, drain and pour them into the sauce with the tuna. Season with the ground pepper, turn off the heat and flavor with the fresh basil leaves. Stir and serve your hot tuna spaghetti!

10) Stewed prawns

Ingredients:
- **Prawns (12 pieces) cleaned 600 g**
- **Peeled tomatoes (cherry tomatoes) 400 g**
- **Water 200 g**
- **Extra virgin olive oil 30 g**
- **Garlic 1 clove**
- **Fresh chili 1**
- **Parsley to taste**
- **Salt to taste**
- **Black pepper to taste**

To prepare stewed prawns, first, start by cleaning the prawns. Clean the prawns leaving the head and tail attached and lay the prawns on a tray. Take the fresh red pepper, extract the internal seeds, and cut it into thin strips. In a pan, heat the olive oil and add a clove of whole peeled garlic and the sliced chili pepper. When the oil is hot, place the prawns in a pan, one next to the other without overlapping them, brown them on both sides for 1 minute. Then add the peeled cherry tomatoes and lengthen the sauce with water. Salt, pepper, cover with the lid, and continue cooking for about 4-5 minutes. Remove the garlic clove with kitchen tongs, mash a portion of the cherry tomatoes with a fork and continue cooking the prawns for about 10 minutes. Wash, dry and finely chop the parsley. When cooked, turn off the heat, flavor the prawns stewed with fresh parsley, and serve them hot.

11) Swordfish rolls

Ingredients:

- **Swordfish 50 g each 4 slices**
- **Basil 8 leaves**
- **Auburn tomatoes 1**

FOR THE STUFFING

- **Chilli powder to taste**
- **1/2 clove garlic**
- **Basil 3 leaves**
- **Green olives 20 g**
- **Capers in salt 20 g**
- **Breadcrumbs 40 g**
- **Auburn tomatoes 2**
- **Extra virgin olive oil 30 g**
- **Salt to taste**

Preheat the oven to 180C. To prepare the swordfish rolls, start chopping the olives and capers with a knife, cut the tomatoes in half, remove the seeds and dice them in a bowl mix the breadcrumbs, capers, chopped olives, chopped garlic clove and tomatoes, half a teaspoon of chili pepper, fresh basil, salt and season with a drizzle of oil. Then take care of the preparation of the swordfish: cut the slices of fish in half, stuff each slice with the filling, about 16 gr of a mixture, fold the edges of the fillet first so as not to let the filling come out, roll it up and stop the rolls swordfish with toothpicks. Cut the tomato into slices and keep them aside, grease an oven dish with oil, arrange the rolls inside and skewer a slice of tomato and a basil leaf on one side, continue in this way with the remaining morsels; before baking, sprinkle the swordfish rolls with a handful of breadcrumbs and season with a drizzle of olive oil. Put in a preheated static oven at 180 ° for just 10 minutes. When the fish rolls turn golden on the surface, take them out of the oven and serve them hot.

12) Octopus In Wet

Ingredients:
- **Clean octopus 800 g**
- **Tomato sauce 310 g**
- **Shallot 1**
- **Garlic 1 clove**
- **Thyme 4 sprigs**
- **Sage 2 leaves**
- **Water 1 l**
- **Extra virgin olive oil to taste**
- **Salt to taste**
- **Black pepper to taste**

Proceed by cleaning the shallot. Then slice it and put it in a bowl, clean the garlic clove and move to the stove. In a large saucepan, heat a round of oil, then add the garlic and shallot. Pour the tomato sauce and turn up the heat, season with salt and add the thyme leaves, the sage, and the water. Heat well until the mixture reaches a boil, dip the octopus tentacles three times. In this way, they will tend to curl properly. Make sure they have assumed the typical curled shape and then immerse them completely. Cover with the lid and cook over medium heat for 50 minutes. For safety, remember to prick the octopus on the inside, where the tooth was, if the fork does not make too much effort to penetrate the pulp, then it is considered cooked. Then sprinkle everything with a minced pepper, and then lift the octopus by moving it on the cutting board, cut it into pieces of the size you prefer and serve with its sauce. Your stewed octopus is ready: enjoy your meal!

13) Pan-fried sea bream

Ingredients:
- **Sea bream 2 clean pieces**
- **Extra virgin olive oil 30 g**
- **Carrots 150 g**
- **Zucchini 150 g**
- **Fresh spring onion 70 g**
- **Garlic 1 clove**
- **Thyme to taste**

Switch to cutting the vegetables: wash and peel the carrots, tick off the ends, and cut them into slices. Wash and check the zucchini, cut them in half lengthwise, divide each half further, and finally cut them into cubes. Finally, wash the onion, remove the base, and cut it into rounds. Pour the oil into a large non-stick pan, add the clove of garlic in the shirt and fry it for a couple of minutes. When the oil is flavored, remove the garlic from the pan and lay the sea bream inside, then add the carrots, zucchini, spring onion, and thyme sprigs, salt, and pepper to taste. Cover the pan with a lid and cook over medium heat for 7 minutes, then turn the sea bream with 2 spatulas, be careful not to break them; cover again with the lid and cook for another 7 minutes. Of course, cooking times may vary depending on the weight of the sea bream you will use. Pan-fried sea bream is ready to be served!

14) Mediterranean salmon fillets

Ingredients:
- **Salmon 800 g**
- **Cherry tomatoes 350 g**
- **Dry oregano 1 sprig**
- **Extra virgin olive oil 30 g**
- **Salt to taste**
- **Garlic 1 clove**
- **Pitted black olives 70 g**
- **Pickled capers 5 g**

Preheat the oven to 180C. To prepare the salmon fillets, start washing the cherry tomatoes, then dry and cut them into 4. Transfer them to a large bowl, add the peeled garlic divided in half, and chop dried oregano. Add the oil, the salt, mix everything and cover with plastic wrap. Leave the cherry tomatoes for about 1 hour at room temperature. After this time, take the salmon steak and extract any bones with a tweezer, and if there is any, remove the skin, then cut into 4 fillets of equal thickness. Pick up the tomatoes, remove the garlic and transfer them to a lightly greased baking dish. Place the salmon fillets on top of the cherry tomatoes, and with a teaspoon, take some cherry tomatoes and arrange them on top of the salmon. Salt, pepper, add the black olives and capers. Bake in a preheated static oven at 180 ° for about 15 minutes. After this time, take out of the oven and serve your Mediterranean salmon fillets while still hot!

15) Sesame tuna

Ingredients:
- **Tuna (4 fillets) 150 g**
- **Black sesame seeds 10 g**
- **White sesame seeds 20 g**
- **Artichokes 4**
- **Lemon juice 1**

FOR THE DRESSING
- **Extra virgin olive oil 35 g**
- **Lemon juice 35 g**
- **Salt to taste**
- **Black pepper to taste**

Start cleaning the artichokes. Prepare a bowl with cold water and squeeze a lemon juice inside: the acidified solution will prevent the clean artichokes from turning black. Cut the part of the stem with the knife, peel the artichokes keeping only the most tender heart, and cut away the leaves' tip with thorns. Remove the most superficial layer of the remaining stalk, which is the most fibrous part, divide the artichokes in half and extract the inner beard. As you clean the artichokes, soak them in the acidulated water you have prepared with the lemon juice. Now prepare the dressing. Squeeze the lemon juice and filter it through a strainer, add a drizzle of olive oil, and whisk emulsify. Salt, pepper, and set aside. Now cut the artichokes into julienne strips, collect them in a bowl and season with half of the seasoning, the rest will serve to season the tuna. In a plate pour the white sesame seeds and the black sesame seeds, mix them. Take the tuna: we

recommend that you make sure that the tuna you have
purchased has been slaughtered; however, we
recommend freezing it for at least 96 hours at -18
degrees, then thawing it before using it in the recipe. Pass
the tuna slices on the seeds to bread them on both sides
as evenly as possible. Heat a non-stick pan and only when
it is hot, lay the tuna fillets in breadcrumbs and cook over
high heat for 1 minute, then turn them over, continue
cooking for another minute. So seared the tuna will be
raw inside, but you can extend the cooking according to
your taste if you like. Once cooked, transfer the fillets to a
cutting board, cut them immediately into slices, and serve
immediately garnishing the sesame tuna with the
remaining dressing and accompanying it with the
artichoke salad.

Chapter 7: Unique dishes

1) Cannellini bean soup

Ingredients:
- Dried cannellini beans 200 g
- Sage sprig 1
- onion 1
- Peeled jar 1
- Extra virgin olive oil of olive, salt and pepper to taste

Soak the beans overnight in plenty of cold water. Drain them and cook them in a pan with salted water until they become tender. Meanwhile, chop the onion with the sage and brown them with olive oil, add the peeled tomatoes and cook for 10 minutes. When the beans are boiled, drain them, keeping some of their water aside and add them to the tomato sauce. Cook for 2/3 minutes, mixing well. Serve as a single dish for lunch or dinner!

2) Meatball soup

Ingredients:
- Minced turkey meat 400 g
- Egg whites 1
- Garlic cloves 2
- Olive oil to taste
- Vegetable broth 1L
- Ground pepper to taste
- Green beans 200g
- Carrots n 4

- **Tomatoes 2**
- **Onions 1**
- **Whole wheat pasta 250g**

Start by washing, cleaning, and cleaning the carrot, onion, 1 garlic, green beans, and tomatoes. Chop the vegetables. In a large saucepan, pour the broth and add all the chopped vegetables. Bring to a boil over high heat and reduce over low heat when you see that the broth begins to boil. Cook until the vegetables have softened. Meanwhile, in a bowl mix the minced meat, the grape white, and the remaining minced garlic. Take a portion of the dough and shape the meatballs by rotating the mixture in your hands. Now take a pot, pour in some olive oil and brown it on the whole surface. To put aside. When the vegetables have softened, take the pasta (the ideal is short pasta or chopped spaghetti to reduce them to 1 cm) and put it in the broth. Season with salt and pepper. After the minutes of cooking the pasta, the soup is ready. Take a bowl and pour the soup, adding the meatballs. Great meal on a cold day!

3) Rice pie

Ingredients:
- **Brown rice g 250**
- **Broccoli g 600**
- **Red onions 1**
- **Eggs 1**
- **2 tablespoons virgin olive oil**
- **2 tablespoons grated Parmesan**
- **Fresh basil**

- **Salt, white pepper**

Preheat the oven to 180 C. Clean and wash the broccoli and put them to boil in a pot full of salt water. When they are tender, drain them and set them aside. In a large pan, brown the finely sliced onion, add the broccoli and cook for a few minutes until the onion wilts. Season with salt and white pepper. Turn off and let cool, apart from boiling the rice in a pan with salted boiling water. Cook for the time written on the package, then drain and keep it aside. Whisk the egg in a bowl with an electric mixer's help, then add the parmesan and chopped basil, a pinch of salt, and the sautéed and chopped broccoli. Add the rice and mix well. Distribute the mixture in slightly greased or non-stick single-dose molds, then inform for 15 minutes. Remove from the oven and serve the hot rice and broccoli flans!

4) Quinoa rocket and parmesan

Ingredients:
- **Quinoa g 70 (for person)**
- **1 carrot**
- **1 celery stalk**
- **1 shallot**
- **1 clove of garlic**
- **A bunch of rocket**
- **Extra virgin olive oil 2 tbsp**
- **Parmesan cheese 50 g**
- **Vegetable broth 500 ml**
- **Salt and pepper**

In a non-stick pan, heat the oil and add minced garlic,

shallot, onion, and celery. Fry very slowly, adding a couple of tablespoons of broth, a little salt, until the vegetables have softened. Add the quinoa (which you have previously rinsed), mix well with the sauté and cook for a minute or two over low heat. Add the boiling broth and cook for about 15 minutes (depends on the cooking time indicated on the package). When the quinoa is cooked, season with salt and add the chopped rocket, grated Parmesan, and pepper pinch. Mix well and serve.

5) Spelled soup

Ingredients:
- **Spelled g 500**
- **Olive oil 1 medium glass**
- **Dark beans 500 g**
- **Carrots 2**
- **Celery 2**
- **Large onions 2**
- **Peeled tomatoes 1/2 Kg**
- **Salt, pepper, chilli pepper**

In a pot full of water, boil beans. Separately chop the onions, carrots, onion, and brown them in a pan with olive oil for about 2/3 minutes, stirring constantly. Add the peeled tomatoes and all the vegetables cut into small pieces; simmer on very low heat for about 15 minutes, adding a part of the bean broth. Add the boiled beans and cook for another 45 minutes; add salt, pepper, and chilli, and then the spelled and continue cooking for 30 minutes on low heat, stirring frequently. Serve hot.

6) Brown rice salad

Ingredients:
- **Brown rice 300 g**
- **Drained tuna in oil 200 g**
- **Auburn tomatoes 150 g**
- **Peas 80 g**
- **Red peppers 75 g**
- **Yellow peppers 75 g**
- **Pitted black olives 80 g**
- **Pickled gherkins 80 g**
- **Chives to taste**
- **Salt to taste**

To make the classic rice salad, put a pan full of salty water on the fire and once it has reached a boil, pour the peas and cook for about 3 minutes. Once this time has elapsed, drain the peas and pour the rice into the same water. Cook the rice 2-3 minutes less than the cooking times indicated on the package. In the meantime, take care of the dressing: wash the peppers, remove the stalk, the seeds, and the internal filaments, cut them first into strips and then into cubes, and place them in a large bowl where you will collect all the other ingredients. Wash and cut the tomatoes in half, dig the pulp with a teaspoon and cut them into cubes, cut the pickled gherkins into rounds and cut the pitted olives in half. When about 2-3 minutes are left from cooking, drain the rice and let it cool by distributing it on a very cold tray to facilitate the rice's cooling. Flavor the dressing with chives cut into small rounds and add the peas and rice that will have cooled in the meantime. Finally, add the crumbled tuna fillets, season with salt, and mix with a spoon. Cover the bowl with plastic wrap and leave it in the refrigerator until ready to serve it so it will be very cold, and the flavors will have mixed.

7)   Vegetable pie

Ingredients:
- **Aubergines Kg 1**
- **Peeled tomatoes 1 jar of 500 g**
- **Onions 200 g**
- **Pepper 1**
- **Mozzarella 300g**
- **Oregano, basil, salt and pepper to taste**

Preheat the oven to 180C. Clean the aubergines, cut them into thin slices and put them on a cutting board, then sprinkle them with salt and leave them for at least 20 minutes so that the water is eliminated inside them. Clean the onion and cut it thinly, also slice the mozzarella. Clean and cut the peppers into strips. In a baking dish, make the first layer with tomatoes (each layer of tomato should be flavored with oregano and basil), then continue with a layer of aubergines and one of the onions. Continue with a layer of tomatoes, then a layer of mozzarella, and an eggplant. The last layer prepare it with all the remaining ingredients plus the pepper. Pass the vegetable pie in the oven at 180 ° C for about an hour. Serve this complete main course hot.

8)   Legumes and cereals soup

Ingredients:

- **Mixed legumes + cereals 500 g**
- **Carrots 2**
- **2 ribs celery**
- **Onions 1**
- **Auburn tomatoes 200 g**
- **Garlic 1 clove**
- **Vegetable broth 1 l**
- **Extra virgin olive oil 3 tbsp**
- **1 sprig rosemary**
- **Thyme 1 sprig**
- **Bay leaf 1 leaf**
- **Sage 1 sprig**

Soak the cereals in cold water in the evening before running the recipe. The following day drain them well, then prepare a mixture with onion, garlic, celery, and carrots. Fry the mince in a pan with oil, then add the drained cereals and legumes, mix for a minute, and then cover with the vegetable broth. Then add the tomatoes, previously peeled and cut into cubes. At this point, add thyme, sage, bay leaf, and form a bunch that you can stop by tying them with a kitchen string and stop at the pot's handle. In this way, they do not scatter in the soup, and you can easily eliminate once cooked. Slowly bring the soup to a boil, season with salt, and then cover the pan with a lid. Cook slowly for at least an hour, adding, if necessary, more vegetable broth so that the soup remains with the right amount of liquid. When cooked, remove the aromatic bunch, adjust if necessary with salt, add a drizzle of extra virgin olive oil and serve in bowls or holsters.

9) Quinoa with vegetables

Ingredients:

- **Quinoa 200 g**
- **Champignon mushrooms 100 g**
- **Red peppers 70 g**
- **Yellow peppers 70 g**
- **Zucchini 150 g**
- **Red onions 100 g**
- **Water 400 g**
- **Extra virgin olive oil to taste**
- **Mint to taste**
- **Salt to taste**
- **Black pepper to taste**

To prepare quinoa with vegetables, start by cleaning the red onions, cutting them in half, and cutting them into thin slices. Also, cut the red pepper in half and scrape away the internal seeds. Then cut it into small cubes, and repeat the same cut also for the yellow pepper. Cut the zucchini into cubes, and finally clean the mushrooms and cut them into slices. Heat a drizzle of oil in a pan and add the onions first. Let them stew slowly, blending with a little water when they begin to brown, and continue cooking for a few more minutes until they are very tender. At that point, add the peppers, mix, and cook a couple of minutes before adding zucchini and mushrooms. Cook all 5 more minutes, seasoning with salt and pepper: your vegetables are ready and beautiful crispy! Now take care of the quinoa: rinse it thoroughly, remove the saponin layer that constitutes the external patina, then heat a little oil on the bottom of a pan and pour the quinoa to toast it. Stir with a wooden spoon to prevent it from sticking, season with salt and continue to cook, cover with the rest of the water: its volume must be twice that of quinoa. As soon as the seeds open to flower and the water has been absorbed, the quinoa is ready: add it to the vegetables. Mix and skip a minute to tie the flavors, then finish with a handful of mint leaves to give the dish its aroma: the quinoa with vegetables is ready to be enjoyed!

10) Chickpea and pumpkin soup

Ingredients:
- **Pumpkin to clean 600 g**
- **Drained pre-cooked chickpeas 400 g**
- **Beets 100 g**
- **Golden onions 100 g**
- **Juniper berries 3 berries**
- **Laurel 2 leaves**
- **Water 1.5 l**
- **Extra virgin olive oil to taste**
- **Salt to taste**
- **Black pepper to taste**

To make the chickpea and pumpkin soup, first, clean the onion and slice it thinly. Time to clean the pumpkin: cut it in half, then empty it of the internal seeds and remove the peel. Cut the pulp first into slices and then into cubes.

Wash the beets and cut them into thin strips. Pour the olive oil into a pan, then add the sliced onion and the juniper berries. Let it cook on a low flame until the onion is soft. At this point, add the pumpkin, brown it over medium heat and then wet with a little water taken from the total dose. Also, add the chickpeas, the chard reduced to strips, salt, pepper, and the rest of the water necessary for cooking. Flavored with bay leaves, mix everything, cover with a lid, and cook on high heat for 15 minutes. After 15 minutes, remove the lid and continue to cook for another 15 minutes. Remove the bay leaves and juniper berries and serve your soup with a drizzle of raw oil and minced black pepper. The pumpkin and chickpea soup are ready to be served.

11) Chickpea shrimp and arugula salad

Ingredients:
- **Clean shrimp 1 kg**
- **Pre-cooked chickpeas 240 g**
- **Rocket 150 g**
- **Pine nuts 30 g**
- **Garlic 1 clove**
- **Paprika 1 tsp**

TO CONDITION
- **Lemon juice 1**
- **Balsamic vinegar 1 tsp**
- **Extra virgin olive oil to taste**
- **Black pepper to taste**
- **Salt to taste**

Start to toast the pine nuts: put them in a pan and toast them for about 5 minutes until golden brown. Heat a drizzle of oil in a pan with the garlic, add the salted prawns, pepper and finally add the paprika. Cook them on high heat for 5 -6 minutes. Once cooked, transfer them to a small bowl to cool. Now drain the pre-cooked chickpeas. In the same pan used for the prawns, heat the chickpeas so that they take on the flavor of the shellfish. Now that all the ingredients are ready, you can compose the salad: Put the washed and dried arugula in a large bowl. Add the chickpeas, prawns, and toasted pine nuts. Mix the salad. Finally, take care of the dressing: prepare an emulsion with oil, salt, pepper. Squeeze the juice of half a lemon, strain it, and add it to the emulsion, finish with a teaspoon of balsamic vinegar. Season the salad with the prepared dressing. Your chickpea shrimp and rocket salad are now ready to be brought to the table!

12) Tuna beans and onion

Ingredients:
- **Drained tuna in oil 120 g**
- **Dried white beans 250 g**
- **Red onions 170 g**
- **Extra virgin olive oil 30 g**
- **Salt to taste**

Put the beans in a bowl full of water and leave them to soak for 12 hours 1. Once this time has passed, drain and rinse them under running water. At this point, transfer them to a pan with water until they are completely covered. Cook the beans for 50 minutes with a lid, checking their cooking from time to time: the beans must be tender, but they must not pulp. When there are 3 or 4 minutes left at the end of cooking, add the salt. Once the beans are cooked, drain them well and let them cool. Switch to the onion: cut the ends, peel it and cut it into very thin slices. Pour the cold beans into a large bowl, add the onion, and the drained tuna. Season with extra virgin olive oil, salt to taste, and mix well with a fork and spoon. Transfer to a serving dish: your tuna beans and onion are ready to be enjoyed!

13) Vegetable and turmeric barley soup

Ingredients:
- **Water 2,5 l**
- **Pearl barley 200 g**
- **Savoy cabbage 300 g**
- **Clean black cabbage 250 g**
- **Clean zucchini 280 g**
- **Dried peas 50 g**
- **Shallot 1**
- **Turmeric powder 15 g**
- **Orange peel 1**
- **Extra virgin olive oil 20 g**
- **Salt to taste**
- **Black pepper to taste**

First, divide the cabbage in half, cut it into strips and rinse it under running water. Do the same with the black cabbage, then reduce it to strips and wash the leaves under the water. Wash, peel, and slice the zucchini into slices, then peel the shallots and slice them. Separately rinse the pearl barley and let it drain in the colander. In a saucepan, heat the olive oil, add the shallot and let it fry over low heat for a couple of minutes. Then add the black cabbage and savoy cabbage, let them dry for a few moments, then pour the water until the vegetables are covered, close with the lid and cook for 2 minutes. At this point, also add the zucchini, pearl barley, and dried peas. Season with the turmeric powder and mix the ingredients, then salt, cover with the lid and cook for 45 minutes, stirring occasionally. If the water decreases during cooking, add more if necessary. Once the soup is ready, serve hot with a drizzle of raw olive oil, a pinch of pepper, and flavored with orange zest to taste. Your barley vegetable and turmeric soup are ready to taste.

14) Whole wheat penne with squid in white wine

Ingredients:
- **Whole Wheat Mezze Penne Rigate 320 g**
- **Clean squid 500 g**
- **Basil to taste**
- **Garlic 1 clove**
- **White wine 30 g**
- **Extra virgin olive oil 10 g**

Proceed by cutting the mantle and tentacles of the squid into strips, so keep aside. In a large saucepan, boil the salted water to taste and cook the pasta, and in the meantime, heat the garlic in a pan with a little extra virgin olive oil. Once browned well, remove it and sauté the squid in a pan for two minutes, occasionally stirring to brown them evenly. Blend everything with the white wine and once it has evaporated, add the pasta al dente and let it flavor with the squid for 3-4 minutes. Take the basil and break it up with your hands, add it in a pan and finally season everything with a spoonful of extra virgin olive oil. Your wholemeal penne with squid in white wine is ready to be served!

15) Sea-scented rice salad

Ingredients:
- **Smoked salmon 50 g**
- **Chives to chop 1 tbsp**
- **Peas 250 g**
- **Prawns 250 g**
- **Cherry tomatoes 8**
- **Clean cuttlefish 200 g**
- **Brown rice 320 g**
- **Parsley 25 g**
- **Extra virgin olive oil 6 tbsp**
- **Clams 500 g**
- **Pitted black olives 60 g**
- **Salt to taste**

Heat a large pan with a couple of tablespoons of olive oil and two cloves of garlic. When it is browned, add the clams, add half of the chopped parsley, and open it. Once the clams are open, strain the cooking liquid and keep it aside, then peel them and put them in a small bowl. Clean the cuttlefish, remove the tentacles and cut the body into strips, then cook them in a pan together with the clam sauce and the remaining parsley, until they have completely absorbed the sauce, it will take about 10 minutes. At this point, peel the prawns and put them to boil in boiling water for about three or four minutes, then drain and keep them aside. Steam the peas and drain when they are still crunchy and a beautiful bright green.

At this point, cook the rice: boil salted water in a large pot and when it has reached a boil, lower the rice, then drain it al dente and place it in a large container with a spoonful of oil to prevent it from becoming sticky. Cut the salmon into julienne strips, quarter the tomatoes, chop the chives, cut the pitted black olives into slices, and put all the ingredients aside. Add the peas with chives to the rice container, then mix. Now add the black olives, the fish (cuttlefish, clams, prawns, and salmon) and the tomatoes. Mix all the ingredients well, season with three tablespoons of extra virgin olive oil and season with salt. Your sea-scented rice salad is ready, serve it on a cold table.

Chapter 8: Side Dish

1) Green beans with raw ham

Ingredients:
- **Boiled green beans 600 g**
- **raw ham 100 g**
- **Onion 1/2**
- **Garlic clove 1**
- **Sprig of rosemary 1**
- **Extra virgin olive oil of olive, salt and pepper to taste**

Take a pot, fill it with water, bring it to a boil, and then boil the beech beans. In the meantime, finely chop the onion and garlic. Boil the green beans, drain them, take a pan and put them on medium heat. Pour the olive oil and let it warm up. When the oil is hot, add the onion and onion. Sauté over medium heat and frequently stir with a wooden spoon. Brown for 3 minutes or until the onion is wilted. Add the ham, green beans, and cook together until the ham becomes slightly translucent. Season with salt and pepper. Serve!

2) Grilled vegetables with yogurt

Ingredients:
- **Medium zucchini 1**
- **Medium aubergine 1**
- **Red bell pepper 1**
- **Yellow pepper 1**
- **Lemon 1**

- **Bunch of chopped parsley 1**
- **Small bunch of chives 1**
- **Extra virgin olive oil of olive, salt and pepper to taste**
- **Skimmed yogurt 1 jar (g 250)**

Take a plate and put it on medium heat. Take the zucchini, cut the ends, and cut them long by making strips of about 0.5 cm. Now take the aubergine, cut the ends, and make round slices about 1cm thick. Take the peppers, cut them in half, and remove the seeds and the filaments inside them. Then cut them into strips. Grease the various vegetables with oil, then place the vegetables on the grilling plate. When the vegetables take on a dark color and have the sign of the plate (or grill) ready, while the vegetables are grilling, take a bowl and put the yogurt, lemon juice, salt, pepper, and oil. Mix everything and add the chopped chives. Put the vegetables on a plate, add the sauce, and mix well. Now they are ready to be served!

3) Zucchini and celery cream soup

Ingredients:
- **1L water**
- **Zucchini 400 g**
- **200g celery**
- **Garlic 1 clove**
- **Pepper 1**
- **Tarragon 1 sprig**
- **Thyme 2 sprigs**
- **Dried oregano 1 pinch**
- **1 tablespoon olive oil**

- **Grated Parmesan 1 tbsp**

Wash and cut the celery and zucchini into small pieces. In a saucepan, bring 1 liter of water to a boil, then add the zucchini, celery, garlic, chilli, oregano, thyme, and tarragon. Cover and cook over low heat for 20 minutes, then season with salt. Once the vegetables are cooked, pour into a container, and with an immersion blender blend all the vegetables adding the Parmesan and a drizzle of olive oil. Serve the cream soup with a fillet of both meat and fish.

4) Fresh spinach and mixed mushrooms

Ingredients:
- **Mushrooms 150g**
- **Olive oil 2 tbsp**
- **2 cloves garlic**
- **Fresh spinach 300 g**
- **Ground pepper and salt to taste**
- **Lemon juice**

Wash, clean the mushrooms, and cut them into coarse pieces. In a pan, over medium-high heat, heat the oil. Add the crushed garlic and sauté for 10 seconds. Add the mushrooms and brown for 2 minutes. Add the spinach, cover, and cook for 2-3 minutes until the spinach wilt. Add the lemon juice, pepper, and serve.

5) Spiced carrots

Ingredients:
- **Carrots 500 g**
- **Laurel 2 leaves**
- **Juniper 3 berries**
- **Black peppercorns 10**
- **Cloves 2**
- **Cardamom 1 pinch**
- **Cinnamon sticks 1**
- **Extra virgin olive oil to taste**
- **Salt to taste**
- **Ground cinnamon to taste**

Start by carefully washing the carrots one by one under running water. Then place them on a cutting board and peel them with a small knife removing the green stem. Take the steamer and fill it with half water (if you don't have it, you can use a large pot and an aluminum colander), heat the water over medium heat, and in the meantime, pour the bay leaves. Then add the peppercorns, juniper berries, cloves, and cardamom seeds. Finally, add the cinnamon stick. When the water starts to quiver, place the steamer basket on top. When the basket is hot, pour the carrots into it. Cover with a lid and cook for about 20 minutes. When the carrots are cooked, transfer them to a serving plate. Salt and pepper to your taste. Finally, pour a drizzle of oil!

6)   Pan-fried artichokes

Ingredients:
- **Artichokes 8**
- **Extra virgin olive oil 50 g**
- **Garlic 1 clove**
- **Salt to taste**
- **Black pepper to taste**
- **Water 150 g**
- **Parsley to taste**
- **Lemon juice**

To prepare pan-fried artichokes, start by cleaning the artichokes. The first important operation to do before starting to clean the artichokes is to rub your hands with lemon to prevent the substances inside this vegetable that oxidize in contact with the air, blacken your hands; alternatively, you can wear some gloves. Always for the same reason, before starting the cleaning of the artichokes, prepare a bowl with cold water in which you will have squeezed the juice of lemon: the acidified solution will prevent the cleaned artichokes from blackening. Once the bowl is prepared, remove the hardest external leaves, cut the stem and eliminate the tip, cutting around 2-3 cm. In addition to having the thorns, this part is the hardest one that will be eliminated even in the artichokes without thorns. Now slightly widen the leaves by exerting a slight pressure towards the outside, eliminating the "beard" with a spoon or a semisphere scoop; if you don't have a scoop, you can use a spoon. Again, remember to dip the artichokes in the acidulated water. In a pan, heat the olive oil with the garlic clove for 1 minute over moderate heat. Drain the artichokes from the acidulated water and squeeze them lightly to remove the excess liquid. Place the artichokes inside the pan with the stem facing upwards. Salt, pepper, add the water. Cover with the lid. Continue cooking for 10 minutes on low heat. Meanwhile, wash and finely chop the parsley. Turn the artichokes and cook for another 20 minutes on the other side. The cooking time may vary according to the artichokes' size, at the end of cooking flavored with chopped parsley and serve the artichokes in a hot pan.

7)   Zucchini salad

Ingredients:
- **Zucchini 800 g**
- **Garlic 1 cloves**
- **Chopped parsley 2 tbsp**
- **Salt to taste**
- **Black pepper to taste**
- **Extra virgin olive oil 40 g**

Wash and peel the zucchini, dry them, and cut them into slices at least 2 mm thick. Put the oil and garlic that you will brown in a non-stick pan, remove it after 5 minutes from the pan and add the zucchini over high heat by covering the pan with a lid and stirring occasionally. A few minutes before the zucchini are ready, add the salt by mixing and the chopped parsley, mix well and serve.

8) Pumpkin sauteed with rosemary

Ingredients:
- Pumpkin pulp 800 g
- 2 sprigs rosemary
- White wine 100 ml
- Garlic 1 cloves
- Extra virgin olive oil 4 tbsp
- Salt to taste
- Black pepper to taste

To prepare the sautéed pumpkin with rosemary, start by cutting the pumpkin into pieces and removing the skin. Then take the pumpkin pulp obtained and cut it into pieces the size of a walnut. Put the oil in a pan, and let the garlic clove brown, which after browning, you can decide to remove or leave in the pan; add the chopped pumpkin and the chopped rosemary and sauté them in a pan until the pumpkin is browned. Take the white wine and sprinkle it on the pumpkin, let it evaporate, then salt it. Continue to cook the pumpkin for about 10 minutes. Pepper to taste and serve immediately!

9) Mixed mushroom salad

Ingredients:
- Mixed mushrooms 800 g
- Extra virgin olive oil 5 tbsp
- Chopped parsley 2 tbsp
- 2 cloves garlic
- Salt to taste

- **Black pepper to taste**

Start cleaning the mushrooms: with a knife, gently scrape the stems, and the lower and upper part of the chapels, removing all the earth. Separate the mushroom chapels from the stems. Now pass a damp cloth on the surface of the mushrooms, removing the remaining soil. Cut the mushroom chapels and stems into slices, then collect them all in a large bowl. Put the oil in a pan and add the crushed garlic that you will brown: add the sliced mushrooms and cook over low heat for 10 minutes. A couple of minutes before the end of cooking, add the salt and pepper, then the chopped parsley. Mix well with a wooden spoon and serve the mushrooms immediately.

10) Cauliflower Salad

Ingredients:
- **Cauliflower 1 medium**
- **Pickled peppers 100 g**
- **Green olives 100 g**
- **Black olives 100 g**
- **Pickled capers 50 g**
- **Cucumbers 50 g**
- **Anchovies (anchovies) in oil 60 g**
- **Extra virgin olive oil 30 g**
- **Red wine vinegar to taste**
- **Salt to taste**

Start by taking the olives: remove the seeds and keep the olives aside. Repeat the operation also for green olives. Then take the gherkins and cut them into thin strips that you will keep aside. Proceed with cleaning the cauliflower. Take the cauliflower, peel it, and remove the hardest final parts. Get the florets that you will boil in a pan with plenty of salted water. When they are cooked but still crunchy, drain them in a bowl filled with ice to stop cooking. Leave it for a few minutes until it is lukewarm, then drain it. Pour the cauliflowers into a large bowl to and add the oil, capers, and green olives, both drained of excess oil. Add the black olives, the pickled peppers rinsed briefly under running water and already cut into thin strips. Finally, add the anchovies. Then pour the gherkins and sprinkle with vinegar. Mix the ingredients well and serve your salad.

11) Baked aubergines and onions

Ingredients:
- **Aubergines 500 g**
- **White onions 2**
- **Pennyroyal 10 leaves**
- **Parsley 1 sprig**
- **Oregano to taste**
- **Basil 10 leaves**
- **Garlic 1 clove**
- **Extra virgin olive oil to taste**
- **Salt to taste**
- **Black pepper to taste**
- **Chilli powder 1 tbsp**

Start by placing the aubergines and onions, washed and dried, in a pan covered with parchment paper. Leave them whole and do not peel them. Cook them in a preheated oven for about an hour at 180 degrees and adjust according to the vegetables' size. When they appear soft and wrinkled, turn off the oven and let them cool. Cut the initial part of the eggplant and peel it. Cut the aubergine into slices about three centimeters high. Then cut each slice into three-four pieces. Take the onions and eliminate the final part. Remove the onion peel, cut the onion in half and deprive it of the heart. Now cut the onion into rather large pieces. At this point, put the pieces of onion and eggplant in a bowl, salt, and pepper, add a clove of garlic without the peel, olive oil, basil pieces, mint, minced parsley, oregano, the chilli. Mix everything so that the odors are well distributed, then remove the garlic clove. Your baked aubergines and onions are ready, and you just have to serve them!

12) Confit tomatoes

Ingredients:

- **Cherry tomatoes 500 g**
- **Garlic 1 clove**
- **Sugar 25 g**
- **Thyme 10 sprigs**
- **Extra virgin olive oil 35 g**
- **Dried oregano to taste**
- **Salt to taste**
- **Black pepper to taste**

Preheat the oven to 140C. Start by washing the cherry tomatoes under running water. Dry them with kitchen paper and place them on a cutting board, then divide all the cherry tomatoes in half. Now arrange the chopped cherry tomatoes on a dripping pan covered with parchment paper with the part of the cut facing upwards.

Then salt and pepper to taste. At this point, prepare the minced garlic and thyme: peel a clove of garlic, peel the sprigs of thyme and then finely chop them together. Once the mince is obtained, pour it over each cherry tomato and add the sugar. Distribute the dried oregano and finally pour a drizzle of oil on each cherry tomato. Put everything in the oven for about 2 hours, until the cherry tomatoes' vegetation water has evaporated and these are not slightly toasted but not dried. At this point, you can taste your confit cherry tomatoes even cold and serve them as a side dish or as a tasty condiment!

13) Tasty lentils

Ingredients:
- **Lentils 400 g**
- **Onions 1**
- **Laurel 3 leaves**
- **Cloves 3**
- **Juniper 4 berries**
- **Extra virgin olive oil 3 tbsp**
- **Black pepper to taste**
- **Vegetable broth 750 ml**
- **Red wine 50 ml**
- **Chunks of raw ham 50g**

Fry the finely chopped onion in a pot with a little oil, on low heat, then add the bay leaves, the juniper berries, and the cloves. Take the raw ham and add it to the onion. When the onion has dried, add the dried lentils. Let it cook for a few minutes, always on low heat, then add the red wine and let it evaporate. Wet the lentils with the broth and continue cooking for at least 50/60 minutes, depending on the lentils' size in a covered pot. Check often that the legumes do not dry out too much: in this case, add a few broth ladles. Finally, add salt and pepper to taste, and serve the flavorful lentils with aromas when they are still hot.

14) Brussels sprouts in a pan

Ingredients:
- **Brussels sprouts 500 g**
- **Speck 120 g**
- **Shallot 40 g**
- **Extra virgin olive oil 50 g**
- **Salt to taste**
- **Black pepper to taste**
- **Vegetable broth 250 g**

Take care of cleaning the sprouts: eliminate the most protruding lower part and remove the outermost leaves. At this point, wash the sprouts under running water, drain, and cut them in half. Keep the sprouts aside and slice the speck, then overlap the slices and cut into strips. At this point, finely chop the shallot and transfer it to a pan where you will have poured the oil. Let it brown on a low flame, stirring often, and only when it is wilted add the strips of speck. Wait about 2-3 minutes, add the Brussel sprouts, salt, and mix everything. Add the vegetable broth and cook covered for about 10-15 minutes. Your pan-fried Brussels sprouts are ready to be enjoyed!

15) Grilled vegetables

Ingredients:
- **Zucchini 300 g**
- **Eggplants 450 g**
- **Peppers 850 g**
- **Tomatoes 200 g**
- **Salt to taste**
- **Black pepper to taste**

Wash all the vegetables under plenty of running water and dry them. Cut the courgettes and aubergines into slices 5 mm thick; take the peppers, remove the upper part, divide them in half, then remove the white filaments and the seeds inside them with a knife. Cut them into rather large cubes and set aside. Remove the stalk of the tomatoes and cut them into 5 mm slices. Once all the vegetables have been cut, put a grill to heat on the fire. When the grill is hot, cook the vegetables a little at a time: distribute the side of the pepper by the side, grill them for 5 minutes, turn them over for even cooking, and then put the courgettes on the fire for 3 minutes and continue with the aubergines for another 3 minutes. Remember to always turn the vegetables over for even cooking. Finally, finish with the tomatoes, cooking them for 4 minutes until they are well grilled. Finally, you can serve your grilled vegetables, seasoning them with olive oil, salt, and pepper.

Chapter 9: Dessert

1)   Baked peaches

Ingredients:
- **Medium, ripe and firm yellow peaches 800 g**
- **Dark chocolate 85% 100 g**
- **Amaretti 80 g**

Preheat the oven to 180C. To prepare the stuffed peaches in the oven, start by rinsing and drying the peaches. Divide each peach in half, then remove the core with a small knife. Also, dig a little the pulp around the hollow of the core. Keep the peaches aside. Now dedicate yourself to the filling: cut the pulp obtained from the peaches and chop it with a knife or using the mixer. Keep it aside. Take the chocolate and finely chop it. Transfer it to a bowl and keep it aside. Take another bowl and crumble the macaroons inside in a coarse way. If you prefer, you can also chop them finely with the help of a mixer. Add the pulp of peaches to the crumbled amaretti. Mix the ingredients with the help of a fork. So also add the chocolate and mix the latter with the ingredients. Finally, arrange the peaches in a lightly buttered baking dish close to each other with the recess facing upwards, preferably without leaving spaces. Fill them with a few spoons of the filling, giving the filling the shape of a small dome. Bake in a preheated static oven at 180 ° C for 60 minutes. After the necessary time, remove the stuffed peaches from the oven and serve them to your guests while still hot!

2) Greek chocolate yogurt mousse

Ingredients:
- **50 g of 85% dark chocolate without minced sugar**
- **490 g of Greek fat-free yogurt**
- **2 tablespoons of sweetener stevia**
- **1 teaspoon of vanilla extract**
- **60 ml of skim milk**
- **180 ml of whipped cream without fat**

Add the chopped chocolate in a microwave-safe bowl. Melt the chocolate completely in the microwave for 1 minute and mix. The chocolate must be melted. In a medium bowl, beat the Greek yogurt with an electric mixer for a few minutes. Add the stevia, vanilla, and milk, and beat a little more, then add the chocolate, a small amount at a time, always mixing it with the mixer's help. When all the chocolate is mixed with yogurt, divide the mousse into 6 portions and add 2 spoons of whipped cream on top of each portion.

3) Fruit and cream cheese dessert

Ingredients:
- **110 g of softened fat-free cream cheese**
- **120 g of fat-free yogurt**
- **1 teaspoon of sugar**
- **half a teaspoon of vanilla**

- **230 g of sliced peaches**
- **225 g of pineapple slices**
- **60 g of grated coconut**

In a small bowl, combine the cream cheese, yogurt, sugar, and vanilla. Use a high speed èlectric mixer, beat until a smooth and compact compound is obtained in a bowl peaches and pineapples. Add the cream cheese mixture and mix. Cover and refrigerate until everything has cooled down. Transfer to a serving plate or bowls. Garnish with grated coconut and serve immediately.

4) Crunchy apple

Ingredients:
- **55 g of brown sugar**
- **30 g of type 0 flour**
- **120 g of oat flakes**
- **30 g softened fat-free margarine**
- **a teaspoon of ground cinnamon**
- **half a teaspoon of nutmeg**
- **5 ml of vanilla extract**
- **5 red apples peeled and sliced**

Preheat the oven to 190 C and grease a 33 x 22 oven tray. In a small bowl, combine brown sugar, flour, oats, margarine, cinnamon, nutmeg, and vanilla. Stir with a fork until the dough is moistened. Pour the dough into the pan and arrange the apples, sprinkle with brown sugar evenly on the top. Cook 30 minutes.

5)   Grilled fruit salad

Ingredients:

For the sugar-free chocolate sauce
- 40 g of cocoa powder
- 180 g of brown sugar
- 80 ml of water
- a teaspoon of vanilla
- a spoonful of canola oil

For grilled fruit
- 1 large wooden skewer soaked in hot water
- 6 large, clean strawberries
- 2 peaches cut into quarters
- half a pineapple cut into thin slices
- 2 slices of watermelon without the zest

Heat a grill or plate. In a small saucepan, mix the cocoa powder, brown sugar, and water. Slowly bring to the boil for one minute over medium heat. Remove from the heat and add the vanilla and canola oil, set aside to cool. Place the strawberries and other fruit on the wooden skewer. Cover all fruit pieces with a spray of canola oil and grill for 3-4 minutes on each outside of the fruit. Do not cook completely. Remove from the grill and allow to cool. Cut the fruit into pieces of equal size and put them in a medium bowl. Store in the refrigerator for 30 minutes. Divide the fruit between six bowls and sprinkle with 1 tablespoon of chocolate sauce. The remaining chocolate sauce can be chilled in a waterproof container and can be used for up to a week.

6) Quinoa pudding

Ingredients:
- **370 ml of skim milk**
- **370 ml of light whipping cream**
- **55 g of brown sugar**
- **1 teaspoon of vanilla**
- **half a teaspoon of ground cinnamon**
- **a pinch of nutmeg**
- **120 g of quinoa**
- **60 g of toasted pumpkin seeds**

Rinse the quinoa under cold water for 2 minutes. Beat the milk, light cream, brown sugar, vanilla, cinnamon, and nutmeg in a medium-sized saucepan, cook over medium heat. Slowly bring to a boil. Once the milk mixture simmers, stir in the quinoa and reduce the heat on low heat. Partially cover the pan and cook for 40 minutes, stirring every 10 minutes. When the quinoa is cooked, add the toasted pumpkin seeds and serve.

7) Chocolate cake

Ingredients:
- **180 g of whole wheat flour**
- **110 g of brown sugar**
- **25 g of bitter cocoa powder**
- **a pinch of salt**
- **1 sachet of baking powder**

- **15 g of vanilla**
- **1 tablespoons of vinegar**
- **60 ml of canola oil**
- **230 ml of water**

Preheat the oven to 175 C. Place the flour, sugar, cocoa powder, salt, and yeast directly in a rectangular pan of approximately 30 x 22. Use a whisk to mix the ingredients. Add the vanilla, vinegar, and oil. Heat the water in the microwave for 3 minutes or until it is boiling. Pour the boiling water slowly and evenly over the ingredients in the pan. Use the whisk to mix everything for 2 minutes. The mixture must be smooth, compact with well blended ingredients. Bake for 25 to 30 minutes or check the cooking with a toothpick that inserted in the center of the cake must come out clean. Allow the cake to cool completely before serving.

8) Sponge cake

Ingredients:
- **4 eggs**
- **80 g sukrin**
- **50 g Lupine flour**
- **10 g Cremor tartar**

Put the whole eggs in a bowl, then place the bowl on top of a pot containing 2 glasses of boiling water, activate the electric mixer and whisk the egg mixture for about 15 - 20 minutes. After the time, remove the bowl from above the pot, add the sweetener to the eggs, whip with the same electric whisk for 10 minutes. Turn off the whips. Add the lupine flour (sieved together with the cream of tartar) and mix with a spatula making circular movements from the bottom upwards, taking care not to disassemble the mixture. Transfer the dough into a mold (35 × 25 cm) and bake in the preheated oven at 190 degrees for 15-20 minutes.

9)   Turmeric plumcake

Ingredients:
- **3 eggs**
- **150 g Type 1 flour**
- **60 g Okara**
- **120 g coconut sugar**
- **35 g Coconut oil**
- **1 Cremor tartar sachet**
- **10 drops Vanilla extract**
- **100 g Carrots**
- **15 g Fresh turmeric**
- **125 g Lactose-free yogurt**

Turn on the oven to preheat it 200 C. Work 3 egg whites for 30 seconds with the electric whisk, add 60 grams of coconut sugar and continue until a well-whipped meringue is obtained. Add the Okara powder, half a sachet of natural yeast, a small amount at a time, and gradually mix with a spatula, always in the same direction and from the bottom upwards. Work with the same electric whisk 3 egg yolks, 60 grams of coconut sugar until a well whipped eggnog is obtained, then add a jar of low-fat yogurt and mix (always in the same direction) with a spatula taking the dough from the bottom upwards tall. Add the carrots and turmeric. Also, add 10 drops of vanilla extract and mix. Add the flour a little at a time, half a sachet of natural yeast and mix. Add the oil and mix. Now transfer the egg yolk mixture (one spoon at a time) to the meringue mixture and gradually mix with the spatula. Transfer the mixture to a 30 x 12 cm oiled and floured cake mold. Place it in the preheated oven for 25 minutes. Try the toothpick, insert it in the cake if it comes out dry the cake is ready

10) Low glycemic index tart

Ingredients:
For shortcrust pastry
- **100 g Hazelnuts**
- **20 g Goji berries**
- **180 g chufa flour**
- **2 eggs**
- **60 g Clarified vegetable butter**
- **60 g Coconut sugar**

For chocolate sauce
- **200 ml Coconut milk**
- **100 g 85% dark chocolate**
- **2 spoons Sukrin**
- **2 tablespoons hazelnut paste**
- **30 g Cocoa butter**

For the coconut cream
- **100 g Coconut milk**
- **50 g Cocoa butter**

Start preparing the shortcrust pastry. Place the hazelnuts,

goji berries in a bowl and blend for 10 seconds. Add chufa
flour, eggs, clarified butter, coconut sugar, and mix for 10
seconds. Put the dough in the fridge for 30 minutes. Now
prepare the chocolate cream: put milk, chocolate,
hazelnut paste, soft cocoa butter, a sweetener in a
saucepan. Turn on the low stove, constantly stir until it
ends with a light boil of at least 2 minutes. Soak the pan
in cold water, stir until cool. Now prepare the whipped
vegetable cream: put the milk in a saucepan, turn on the
low stove and bring it to a boil, turn off the stove and add
to the cocoa butter and sweetener. Leave to cool and
work with the whisk until the mixture turns into whipped
cream. Take the pastry from the fridge and spread it
between 2 sheets of parchment paper. Place it in a tart
mold (about 20 cm in diameter). Remove the excess
pastry. Bake the base in the preheated oven at 190 ° for
10 - 15 minutes. Remove from the oven and let it cool for
5 minutes. Spread the chocolate cream on the cold base.
Garnish with whipped coconut cream.

11) Roll stuffed with chestnut cream

Ingredients:
- **4 eggs**
- **90 g coconut sugar**
- **80 g wholemeal flour**
- **3 tablespoons carbonated water**
- **8 g Cremor tartar**
- **For the chestnut cream**
- **500 g Chestnuts**
- **360 g Coconut milk**

Put the chestnuts to boil about 20 - 30 minutes with

plenty of water and a drizzle of oil, then drain and peel them. Chop them roughly then cook them together with the milk for another 20 - 30 minutes. In the end, blend them with a robot with blades and create the cream. Prepare the cookie dough: work the egg whites with the electric whisk. Work with the same whisk yolks, coconut sugar dissolved in the water. Add flour, cream of tartar. Finish the process with two rounds of whips then turn off. Transfer the whipped egg whites to the yolk mixture and mix with a spatula. Transfer the mixture to a baking tray covered with parchment paper (40 x 30 cm). Bake at 190 degrees for 7 minutes. Once the cookie dough is baked, you can turn it over on a sheet of parchment paper then remove the sheet of parchment paper that is now towards you. Spread the chestnut cream on the biscuit dough then roll up.

12) Lemon sorbet

Ingredients:
- **300 ml water**
- **200 ml egg whites**
- **100 ml lemon juice**
- **Stevia (a tip of a teaspoon)**

Put the water in a saucepan, egg whites (lightly beaten with a fork), lemon juice, stevia. Bring to a boil then cook for 1 minute. Turn off the stove, immerse the pot in cold water. When the mixture is well cooled, place it in a silicone container. When the mixture is well frozen, pass it in a food processor with blades, operate it until a creamy and hard mixture is obtained. Serve it right away!

13) Cherry cheesecake

Ingredients:
For yogurt mousse
- **15 g Gelatine sheets**
- **5 tbsp milk**
- **250 g Yogurt (with cherry)**

For ricotta mousse
- **500 g Ricotta**
- **1/2 teaspoon pure Stevia**
- **3 tablespoons Bitter cocoa powder**

To garnish
- **500 g Cherries**
- **1 tablespoon Stevia**

For the base
- **160 g Sugar free biscuits**
- **125 g Mascarpone light**

Let's start from the base: blend with a robot with blades 160 g of biscuits, then transfer them to a bowl, add the mascarpone and mix with a spatula to create a homogeneous mixture. Spread the mixture on the bottom of a mold with an opening circle and level it with a spoon's back. Transfer the mold to the fridge. For the yogurt mousse: soak the jelly for 10 minutes. Then squeeze it and dissolve it in the 5 spoons of warm milk. Add it to the mixed yogurt and transfer the mixture to the fridge. For the ricotta mousse: in a bowl, add the ricotta, 1/2 teaspoon of Stevia, 3 spoons of bitter cocoa. Stir to create a homogeneous mixture. Add the 2 mousses and mix with a spatula until the two compounds are mixed. Put the mousse obtained in the freezer 15 minutes. In the meantime, prepare the cherries: wash and dry the cherries, then toss them. Put them on a sheet of parchment paper then sprinkle them with 1 tablespoon of Stevia. Roll them and leave them aside. Pour the mousse onto the base, level it, and put it in the freezer for 30 minutes. After the time, take back the mold, then open the hinge and remove the metal circle. Pour all the cherries in the center of the cake, then sprinkle a little more with Stevia, and the cherries.

14) Pears Cake

Ingredients:
- **1 Pear 350 g**
- **80 g Soft wheat flour**
- **50 g Coconut sugar**
- **40 g Coconut milk**
- **8 g Creamy tartar natural yeast**
- **2 eggs**
- **Half lemon juice + grated peel**
- **1 tablespoon vanilla extract**
- **30 g grated coconut**

First of all, oil a cake pan (diameter 20 cm) and cover the bottom with a parchment paper disk. Then, halfway through the work, turn on the oven at 190 °. Prepare and weigh all the ingredients. The pear cut into not too large pieces in a bowl mix, a teaspoon of coconut sugar, juice and grated peel of half a lemon, vanilla, and mix. In another bowl, put 2 egg whites, then whisk them with the electric mixer. In another bowl, put 2 yolks, 1 tablespoon of coconut milk and work with an electric whisk for a few seconds, add all the remaining coconut sugar, and continue working with the whisk until the mixture has tripled in volume. Add the flour (1 tablespoon at a time) together with the sifted natural yeast, alternate with a drizzle of coconut milk, and with each addition, give two turns with a spoon without removing the volume of the dough. Add the pears with all the bottom liquid. Give two turns with the spoon then add the beaten egg whites and mix. Transfer the mixture to the pan and bake at 190 degrees for 30 minutes.

15) Strawberry ice cream

Ingredients:
- **400 g Strawberries**
- **250 g Light ricotta**
- **15 g Stevia**
- **1 tablespoon lemon juice**

Wash and dry the strawberries on kitchen paper. Put them in a container of an immersion mixer, add the lemon juice, and blend a few moments. Add stevia, ricotta, then operate the mixer again to create a velvety mixture. Transfer the strawberry and ricotta mixture to the freezer for about 1 hour. After the necessary time, you can enjoy it on a hot summer day.

Chapter 10: Sauces & Condiment

1) Salsa At Nuts

Ingredients:
- **Walnuts 160 g**
- **Extra virgin olive oil 70 g**
- **Garlic 1 clove**
- **Pine nuts 20 g**
- **Grated Parmesan 30 g**
- **Skimmed milk 160 g**
- **Marjoram 4 g**
- **Wholemeal bread crumbs 30 g**

To prepare the walnut sauce, first, take a pan with high edges, pour the water, and bring it to the boil. When the water is boiling, pour the kernels for at least 5 minutes. This operation will allow you to deprive them of the external skin more easily afterwards. Then drain the kernels with the help of a colander and lay them on a clean tea towel so that they dry and cool. In the meantime, take a bowl with high sides and pour the breadcrumbs to which you will add the milk. Mix the crumb with milk so that it can moisten well. When the breadcrumbs have softened, pour the bowl with the bread over a narrow mesh strainer placed on top of a small bowl to drain the excess milk and, if necessary, apply light pressure with a spatula. Collect the excess milk and set aside. Now take the warm kernels and remove the outer skin. Then put them in a mixer together with bread previously soaked in milk and pine nuts. Then add also garlic, marjoram, and grated cheese. Operate the blender and gradually add the oil and milk kept aside to make your walnut sauce creamier and denser. Season with salt and pepper. When you have obtained a nice homogeneous mixture, your walnut sauce will be ready to flavor dishes!

2)   Fresh tomato sauce

Ingredients:
- **Auburn tomatoes 1,2 kg**
- **Extra virgin olive oil 3 tbsp**
- **Salt to taste**
- **Basil 8 leaves**

When you buy the tomatoes from the sauce, check them one by one, eliminating the bad, stained, or dented ones. Remove the stalks and wash them very well, then dry them. Cut each tomato in two halves, and remove the green part of the petiole from each. Squeeze the two halves of the tomato in a bowl or sink so that all the seeds come out. Put the sauce tomatoes in a steel pot 8, which you will place on a low heat covered by the lid; let the tomatoes cook, turning them from time to time until they are wilted and unravel. At this point, pass the tomatoes with the vegetable mill, converging the sauce in a bowl; once you have passed all the tomatoes, pour the pass into a smaller steel pot that you will put on the fire. Add the salt and oil to the sauce and cook over high heat to the desired density, then turn off the heat and add the whole or coarsely chopped basil to the sauce by hand.

3) Guacamole

Ingredients:
- **Ripe avocado 1**
- **Green hot pepper 1**
- **Auburn tomatoes 1**
- **Extra virgin olive oil 20 g**
- **Lime juice 10 g**
- **Shallot 10 g**
- **Black pepper 1 pinch**
- **Salt up to a pinch**

Cut the avocado in half lengthwise, then sink the knife's blade into the core and pull to extract it easily. Carve the pulp with a knife to extract it more easily with a spoon; collect it in a small bowl. Then cut the lime in half and squeeze it to obtain the juice, be poured on the avocado pulp; Then season with salt and pepper, and mash the pulp with a fork. Keep aside, then clean and finely chop the shallot, then wash, dry, and slice the tomato 10: made from the cubes' slices. Then tick the chili pepper, empty it of its seeds and cut it into strips, then also diced. Then in the bowl with the crushed avocado pulp, pour the chopped shallots and the diced tomatoes. Also, add the chili pepper and the oil, mix, and season again with salt and pepper if necessary. Your guacamole sauce is ready to be enjoyed!

4)

5) Lentils cream

Ingredients:

- **Lentils 250 g**
- **2 ribs celery**
- **Carrots 2**
- **White onions 1**
- **Small potatoes 2**
- **2 cloves garlic**
- **Zucchini 2**
- **Laurel 2 leaves**
- **Cumin 1 tsp**
- **Cloves 2**
- **Extra virgin olive oil 2 tbsp**
- **Salt to taste**
- **Boiling water 2,5 l**

Soak the lentils in cold water for at least 12 hours. After the soaking time, start cleaning the vegetables, and cut the carrots into cubes, after peeling them, the celery and the zucchini. Heat the oil with the garlic in a saucepan with high sides; finely chop the onion, add it to the pan, stew it gently, and add all the vegetables except the lentils. Cook for about 10 minutes on low heat mixing them with a wooden spoon; when they are tender, add the lentils well drained from the soaking water, the bay leaves and the cloves, also pour the cumin powder and season with salt; lastly, pour the hot water, or vegetable broth, bring gently to a boil, cover with a lid and cook over low heat for about 2 hours, or until the lentils are well cooked and tender (but not unmade); if necessary, add more water if the soup dries out too much. Before serving, remove the bay leaves and possibly also the cloves and put in a blender container. With an immersion blender, blend the soup until a smooth and homogeneous mixture is obtained. Excellent to serve on whole wheat bread croutons as an appetizer or as an accompaniment to meat or fish dishes.

6)   Pistachio pesto

Ingredients:
- **Shelled pistachios 200 g**
- **Grated cheese 35 g**
- **½ lemon zest**
- **½ clove garlic**
- **Extra virgin olive oil 100 ml**
- **Water 100 ml**
- **Basil 3 leaves**
- **Salt to taste**
- **Black pepper to taste**

To make the pistachio pesto, start by placing a pot full of water on the fire, bring it to the boil, pour the shelled pistachios, cook for 5 minutes, or the time needed to soften the peel then drain the pistachios. Remove the pistachio peel and collect them in a small bowl. Transfer the pistachios to a mixer, pour the olive oil, the grated cheese, the basil leaves, half a clove of garlic and the grated zest of half a lemon. Operate the blades for a few moments and then pour the water, salt, pepper, and operate the blades again, blend the mixture until obtaining a homogenous cream.

7) Sicilian pesto

Ingredients:
- **Auburn tomatoes 500 g**
- **Pine nuts 50 g**
- **Extra virgin olive oil 150 ml**
- **Garlic 1 clove**
- **Basil 1 bunch**
- **Parmesan cheese DOP to be grated 100 g**
- **Light ricotta 150 g**
- **Salt to taste**
- **Black pepper to taste**

Start by carefully washing the tomatoes and dividing them in half. Once divided, eliminate the internal part and squeeze them to eliminate the seeds and excess juice. Then wash the basil leaves under running water and, after draining them, dry them with a cloth. At this point, pour the tomatoes into a mixer, add the washed and dried basil leaves and the pine nuts. Peel a clove of garlic, divide it in half and add it to the mixture together with the grated Parmesan and ricotta. Salt and pepper to taste. After adding all the ingredients, pour the oil and operate the mixer at low speed to check the creaminess's desired degree. You can decide whether to obtain a more or less creamy mixture. When the pesto has reached the right consistency, check if you still need salt and pepper. Now the Sicilian pesto is ready to enrich and color your pasta!

8)   Black olives pate

Ingredients:
- **Black olives 200 g**
- **Extra virgin olive oil 45 g**

To prepare the olive patè, start by pitting the olives one by one, place them in the blender and blend them until you obtain a homogeneous mixture. Add the extra virgin olive oil flush, until you get a soft and sufficiently compact cream. Your pate is ready to be served. You can enjoy it on crispy croutons: to prepare them, simply slice the bread, place it on a dripping pan lined with parchment paper, sprinkle it with a little oil and toast it on the oven in grill mode for 2 minutes, turning it halfway through cooking to make it toast evenly. You can spread the black olive patè on hot bread with a drizzle of oil cooked in the oven until it takes on a golden color.

9)   Chilli cream

Ingredients:
- **Spicy fresh chili 300 g**
- **Garlic 1 clove**
- **Extra virgin olive oil 90 g**
- **Coarse salt 140 g**

Wash the chillies under running fresh water, clean them: with a small knife, remove the stalk, then open them in half lengthwise; remove the pulp and seeds and then keep the chillies aside. Sprinkle a tray lined with a dry tea towel with 70 g of salt and place the cleaned chillies side by side. Once spread, sprinkle the entire surface with the rest of the salt you have preserved, distributing it evenly over all the chillies; when you are finished, cover everything with another cloth or with a tray. Leave the peppers covered for 2 days so that they lose the water, then with the help of a brush, carefully remove the excess salt from each chili pepper. After this operation, take the garlic clove, cut it in half, and remove the soul with a knife. Place the cleaned peppers in the bowl of a chopper together with the clove of garlic, add the oil flush and then blend until obtaining a smooth and homogeneous cream. At this point, you can decide whether to consume the chili cream immediately or keep it for a long time: in this case, sanitize an airtight jar, then fill it with the cream and close the cap.

10) Garlic sauce

Ingredients:
- **4 cloves garlic**
- **Peeled almonds 50 g**
- **Extra virgin olive oil 250 ml**
- **Chopped parsley 2 tbsp**
- **White wine vinegar 2 tbsp**
- **Salt to taste**
- **Black pepper to taste**
- **Potatoes 80 g**

Prepare the garlic sauce, wash the potato well, and boil it with all the peel in salted water; when cooked, drain it and let it cool. Once cold, peel it and cut it into wedges. Clean the garlic and put it in the mixer, add the peeled almonds, the parsley, the vinegar, the potatoes, salt, pepper, and blend everything by adding the oil little by little. Once a thick cream is obtained, the garlic sauce will be ready to be served with your dishes.

11) Mint pesto

Ingredients:
- **Mint (about 50 leaflets) 10 g**
- **Pine nuts 40 g**
- **Extra virgin olive oil 50 ml**
- **Salt to taste**
- **Black pepper to taste**

Start by removing the mint leaves from the twigs, then wash them under running water and let them drain in a colander. Finally, dry them well with a paper towel. Take a mixer to chop and place the mint leaves, pine nuts, salt, pepper, and a drizzle of oil inside. Run the mixer for a couple of minutes until the ingredients are chopped then add the remaining oil gradually until you get a creamy consistency. If necessary, adjust again with salt and pepper, and keep the mint pesto sauce in the refrigerator until ready for use.

12) Citronette

Ingredients:
- **Lemon juice 40 g**
- **Extra virgin olive oil 60 g**
- **Salt 1 pinch**
- **Black pepper to taste**

Start squeezing the juice of one lemon and filter it with a strainer. Pour the juice into a large bowl. Also, add the salt and begin to emulsify with a whisk. You can also use a mixer if you prefer. When the salt is completely dissolved, also add the pepper and continue to mix. Then add the oil. Continue to quickly emulsify the ingredients to obtain a homogeneous and slightly dense citronette. When the ingredients are well blended, the citronette is ready to be used in your meat, fish, and side dish preparations!

13) Sugar-free cake cream

Ingredients:
- **100 g Skimmed milk**
- **10 g icing sukrin**
- **1 g Tara or Guar flour**
- **35 g Powdered milk**

Combine the powdered milk, sukrin, tara flour in a bowl and mix well. Put the milk in a tall, narrow container. Work it with the electric whips for 20 seconds, and while the whips are in action, add all the powders at once. Continue to work with the electric whisks at maximum speed by folding the container on one side. Without dropping the cream and the whips, make them work horizontally. Continue to work with the whisk at maximum speed until everything becomes whipped cream.

14) Coffee cream

Ingredients:
- **500 g Skimmed milk**
- **5 egg yolks**
- **80 g sukrin**

- **65 g lupine flour**
- **Half a teaspoon Tara flour**
- **2 teaspoons Soluble ginseng coffee**

Work with electric whisk yolks, sukrin for about 1 minute. Set aside half a glass of milk, add the rest to the yolks little by little alternating with the sifted lupine flour, and the instant coffee always with the whips in motion. When the mixture is amalgamated, transfer the pan to the stove and cook until boiling, stirring constantly. Then turn off the stove. Now take the milk aside, beat it with the electric whisk, and at the same time, add the tare flour. When the milk takes on the appearance of smooth and thick cream, it is ready. Immediately transfer the tare cream to the coffee cream. Mix with a spatula making rotational movements from the bottom upwards until the cream takes on a dense and smooth appearance. Cover with contact film and immerse the pan in cold water. When the cream has cooled down, it is ready to be used to fill a cake, a cake, cream puffs, or a tart (in any case always on bases prepared following the insulin resistance diet.

15) Custard

Ingredients:
- **500 ml Milk**
- **80g sukrin**
- **65 g lupine flour**
- **5 egg yolks**
- **Half a teaspoon Tara flour**

Work with electric whisk yolks and sukrin for about 1

minute. Set aside half a glass of milk, add the rest to the yolks little by little alternating with the sifted lupine flour with the whisk in motion. When the mixture is amalgamated, transfer the pan to the stove and cook until boiling, constantly stirring with a spatula. Then turn off the stove. Now take the milk aside, beat it with the electric whisk, and at the same time, add the tare flour. When the milk takes on the appearance of smooth and thick cream, it is ready. Transfer the tare cream to the lupine flour cream immediately. Mix with a silicone spatula making rotational movements from the bottom upwards until the cream takes on a dense and smooth appearance. Cover with contact film and immerse the pan in cold water. When the cream has cooled down, it is ready to use to fill a cake, a cake, cream puffs, or a tart, however, always on bases prepared following the diet of insulin resistance.

16) Rocket and hazelnut pesto

Ingredients:
- **150 g Rocket**
- **80 g Hazelnuts**
- **30 ml Extra virgin olive oil**
- **1 pinch Himalayan salt**
- **1 clove of garlic**

First of all, remove the yellow leaves and the root part of the rocket, then immerse it in cold water and rinse it well several times. Now collect the leaves in a perforated bowl and drop the excess water, then spread all the rocket on a clean (possibly uncolored) kitchen cloth, roll up and squeeze hard until no more liquid comes out. With a simple mixer with blades, insert all the glass ingredients and operate at maximum speed. The arugula and hazelnut pesto are ready; you can use it immediately, for example, on croutons, or vegetables, meat or fish.

Conclusion

The role of insulin is to allow the body's cells to incorporate sugars, to be used as fuel or stored as body fat. Insulin resistance, if left untreated, can lead to risks and complications, including type 2 diabetes, heart, kidney, and liver problems. So it is important to completely change your lifestyle associated with a proper diet. The main reason for this problem is the excessive blood glucose level. The treatments in the initial phase of insulin resistance consist of the correct intake of food, exercise, and following a healthy diet, trying to reduce weight. In addition, carrying out a proper medical check-up will help you find out how serious the problem is. Consult your family doctor and listen to treatment recommendations and precautions. This is the first step you need to take to treat insulin resistance. In this book, a series of healthy and organic recipes are mentioned that will finally help you enjoy good food without promoting the risk of insulin resistance.

PCOS
Cookbook

Introduction

Polycystic ovary syndrome (PCOS) is one of the most common hormonal disorders in women; it affects 5-10% of it in fertile age. It would not be surprising if this number increased since then, based on the increased prevalence of sedentary and stressful lifestyles and endocrine disruptors in personal care products and food supplies. PCOS is not a real disease, and it is not severe, in the sense that it does not endanger your general health and, indeed, not your life. But this condition of hormonal imbalance still compromises the quality of your life as a woman, and above all, it is harmful to your fertility. A polycystic ovary has the characteristic of filling with microscopic fluid-filled cysts, which prevent follicles from producing ovulation during the ovulation phase. Polycystic ovary syndrome involves hormonal imbalance, which in the long run, can create problems by changing the physical appearance of those who suffer from it, which in turn can cause emotional distress and lead to depressive forms. Not all patients will have the same symptoms. The symptoms of PCOS can also be shown mildly, as some women find they suffer from it only when the woman is unable to conceive. Although the first thing to do is contact your family doctor, for the most appropriate treatment, in this guide, you will find everything you need to know about the possibilities of treatment, prevention, and many useful tips for a correct lifestyle. You will also find numerous recipes designed specifically for all women who suffer from this problem.

Chapter 1: What is PCOS?

Polycystic ovary syndrome or PCOS also called ovarian polycystic, Stein-Leventhal syndrome, or hyperandrogenic anovulation, is a complex of symptoms resulting from a hormonal imbalance. In women of reproductive age, it is one of the major endocrine disorders that affect women, especially in the pubertal period and is characterized by ovulatory dysfunctions: ovarian enlargement, hyperandrogenism, and the presence of ovarian cysts. Excessive hormone production, together with the absence of ovulation, can cause infertility. In PCOS, many follicles never reach complete development, thus causing ovulation problems, sometimes conditions of infertility linked to chronic anovularity, irregular menstrual cycles, or, again, overweight and hirsutism. Etiology is still controversial today. It can be said that the polycystic ovary is the expression of a complex functional alteration of the reproductive system given by the increase in male hormones in women.

Types of PCOS

Although there is a tendency to talk about PCOS in a generic way, you should know that the scientific community has identified 4 types of PCOS, which are:

Classic PCOS

This group includes women who experience cycle disorders, signs of hyperandrogenism but do not have a polycystic ovary.

PCOS Ovulatory

When polycystic ovaries and signs of hyperandrogenism occur, but regular ovulatory cycles. Women with ovulatory PCOS generally have intermediate levels of androgens, insulin, atherogenic fats, and a prevalence of metabolic syndrome.

Non-hyperandrogenic PCOS

It is based on the presence of ovulatory disorders and polycystic ovary, the signs of hirsutism and hyperandrogenism are absent. This group is described as non-hyperandrogenic PCOS. In most of the studies conducted, it was found that endocrine and metabolic dysfunctions were less pronounced in these women, and metabolic syndrome was also less present.

PCOS Complete

The women who fall into this group present what we might call complete PCOS. These are women who experience all 3 of the symptoms described above. This is also the most common type of PCOS and the one associated with major health risks. PCOS women in this group are more likely to also have insulin resistance and overweight or obesity. In particular, women in this group have a higher prevalence of abdominal fat.

Causes

PCOS is a multifactorial syndrome, but the exact causes of the metabolic and hormonal decompensation that determines it are the subject of scientific studies. What we know for sure is that:

- Genetic predisposition could be one of the causes of PCOS. A study conducted by the University of Alabama showed that in 24% of women with PCOS, the mother also suffered from the syndrome. Also, 32% of women had a sister with the same conditions. Women who are familiar with PCOS have a higher risk of developing the same metabolic changes. However, there is not a single genetic factor involved in PCOS. In fact, for the syndrome to manifest itself, multiple genes and mechanisms contribute.

- Women who develop the syndrome secrete an abnormal amount of androgenic hormones (which in turn are associated with hirsutism, acne, and hair loss), which prevent ovarian follicles from producing the egg to be fertilized every month. And this is the reason why women with polycystic ovary syndrome have difficulty getting pregnant. Indeed, suffering from PCOS is a major cause of female infertility. PCOS is associated with elevated insulin levels and subsequent metabolic syndrome. It means that although the pancreas of women with polycystic ovaries produces enough insulin to metabolize the ingested carbohydrates (i.e., food carbohydrates, the macronutrients that provide energy to the body's cells), in reality, this does not happen. Therefore it is necessary to increase the concentration of insulin for achieving the same result. But too much-circulating insulin is associated with overweight, hypercholesterolemia, hyperglycemia, and often hypertension. Furthermore, it is still possible that sugar metabolism is jammed, and a propensity for type 2 diabetes may bind to PCOS.

- Polycystic ovary syndrome is often linked to a condition of sub inflammation. This occurs when the body's immune system puts too many antibodies into circulation as if it were a little hyperactive. This, in turn, stimulates the ovaries to produce more androgenic hormones than necessary.

- Despite having gynecological repercussions, it is good to clarify that polycystic ovary syndrome mainly derives from an insulin hormone dysfunction, which performs the important task of regulating blood glucose levels. Up to 80% of women with PCOS have insulin resistance: the body does not use insulin properly and cannot maintain glucose levels stable. Since the available insulin doesn't work as it should, the body tends to produce more. This malfunction causes an increase in the production of androgens (male hormones), such as testosterone. For this reason, acne and hirsutism are among the most common symptoms of polycystic ovary syndrome.

- Overweight women with PCOS can have a form of insulin resistance caused by bad eating habits and poor physical activity. The role of nutrition in onset, as well as in the treatment of PCOS, is increasingly being studied and studied. Many scholars have even speculated that ovarian polycystic may be caused by bad eating habits during the first years of life, to underline the importance that the right diet has for the physiological well-being of the body.

Symptoms

It must be said that this syndrome can affect 15 to 45 years, with a "peak" between 20 and 30 years. If, therefore, you find yourself in this age range and want to understand if the problems you encounter in your reproductive life or your monthly cycle are attributable to a polycystic ovary, try to consult the long list of possible symptoms of PCOS and tick those in which you find yourself:

- **Irregular menstrual cycle**: Generally, women with polycystic ovary syndrome go from having very few menstruations per year, with little flow, to phases in which, on the contrary, they suffer from hypermenorrhea (too abundant menstruation). In some cases, the cycle stops completely with the total absence of menstruation for more than three months (amenorrhea). In less severe cases, the cycle can still be altered; an example is intervals of over 35 days between menstruation and the next or less than 21 days.
- **Hirsutism**: Excessive hair, especially in areas of the body normally hairless in women, such as the face, chest, or back, is a sign of hyper testosterone production. This symptom is somewhat indicative of PCOS because it affects about 70% of young women with polycystic ovaries.**Acne**: Even the overproduction of sebum that causes acne, or the formation of inflamed pimples full of pus, depends on stimulation beyond the norm of androgenic hormones. In general, the skin appears oily and tends to be impure.
- **Alopecia**: Hair loss with hair loss in a young woman can be a symptom of PCOS because this defect has a lot to do with excessive testosterone production.

- **Overweight**: The alteration of the metabolism that occurs in PCOS sufferers also involves the tendency to gain weight, and vice versa. The fat cells, in turn, stimulate hormonal production and predispose to further accumulation of fat. Also, slowed metabolism makes the weight loss process more difficult and slow. For this reason, as we will see, it is recommended to follow a controlled low-calorie diet. Typically, polycystic ovary syndrome leads to the formation of adipose panniculus in areas such as the neck or the arms. Overweight can lead to obesity, which represents both a risk factor and a complication of PCOS.

- **Skin spots, darker skin**. These discolorations are commonly seen in the folds of the neck and arms.

However, if you believe you have more of these symptoms, you should go to a specialist in gynecology or endocrinology to carry out the diagnostic investigations necessary to find out if the cause of your symptoms is a PCOS.

PCOS diagnosis

Since polycystic ovary syndrome is mainly a hormonal disorder, treatment will also go in that direction. Especially for younger girls, hormonal preparations are available that inhibit the hyperproduction of testosterone and other androgenic hormones. However, we consider that a condition like PCOS is not completely reversible, and the therapies are mainly aimed at reducing its symptoms and preventing more serious complications. But before we get to therapy, let's start with the diagnosis. The process involves several steps, including:

- **Specialist endocrinological examination:** This physical examination of the patient allows to evaluate the physical symptoms determined by PCOS, and to detect the possible presence of acne and excess hair, to measure the waist and pressure.

- **Pelvic ultrasound:** Indispensable for viewing the state of the ovaries and identifying microcysts.
- **Hormonal dosages and blood tests for lipid profile and blood sugar:** Through blood tests, it is possible to measure of male hormones's concetration and evaluate the general conditions associated with the polycystic ovary, including excessive production of insulin, hyperglycemia, and hypercholesterolemia. Sometimes dosages are also made for thyroid hormones, in particular TSH, often altered in women with PCOS.

Chapter 2: Treatments, risks and complications

If neglected, polycystic ovary syndrome can cause serious health problems, such as diabetes, cardiovascular disorders, and even cancers, such as endometrial cancer. Women with PCOS mature many microcysts in their ovaries, which in themselves are not serious, but involve a hormonal imbalance that, in the long run, can create the problems just mentioned. Also, this syndrome that causes abnormal increases in testosterone and other male hormones in fertile women can change the appearance of those who suffer from it, leading to imperfections such as hirsutism, acne, overweight, which in turn can cause emotional distress and lead to depressive forms. Now let's go to the possible treatments for PCOS.

Treatments

Having made the diagnosis, what are the possible treatments? The options currently available are the following:

Pharmacological therapy

- **Drugs reduce the production of androgenic hormones, including**: flutamide, drospirenone, dienogest, chlormadinone, cyproterone acetate. These active ingredients also positively influence the symptoms by reducing hirsutism, improving the aesthetics of the skin and hair. But be careful, the doctor must establish the dosages and constantly monitor to avoid dangerous side effects.

- **Hormonal contraceptives to rebalance female hormone levels:** These devices, of course, are especially indicated for very young women who do not seek pregnancy and in the absence of vascular complications.
- **Metformin**: It is a drug indicated to reduce excessive insulin levels in the blood and therefore help fight metabolic syndrome and diabetes.
- **Medicines for ovarian stimulation:** Clomiphene, Serophene, synthetic gonadotropins, etc., are molecules capable of effectively stimulating ovulation and therefore helping women with PCOS who are looking for a pregnancy, to become pregnant.

All these treatments should only be adopted after consulting your doctor. However, drug therapy is not the only way to reduce the symptoms that PCOS entails, regularize the menstrual cycle, and combat infertility. It is also essential to adopt behavioral rules that help the body to return to balance.

Lose weight

We have seen how weight gain is one of the main risk factors for PCOS, so one of the first suggestions that doctors provide to women who suffer from it is precisely to try to lose weight. To do this, it is necessary to avoid do-it-yourself and have a personalized diet program prescribed by a nutritionist expert in nutrition suitable for polycystic ovary syndrome. Reducing the overall calorie intake, increasing the intake of fibers and antioxidants contained in fruit, vegetables, legumes, and whole grains and drastically cutting the consumption of simple sugars are the cornerstones of a healthy and balanced diet.

Doing motor activity

Making your life more dynamic, for example, by practicing a sport or at least doing more walking, jogging, swimming, etc. is essential if you want to stimulate the metabolism and reduce the waistline. Cholesterol levels, blood pressure, and insulin production will significantly benefit.

Proper nutrition

Scientific studies have shown that one of the first steps towards PCOS treatment is to adopt a healthy vision style. It means weight control through a specific nutrition program for PCOS. Be careful, because it's not just about losing weight. Many women who suffer from PCOS do not need to lose weight. Here we talk about the PCOS diet, that is, a nutritional program with specific foods to reduce the body's inflammatory condition and keep hormonal imbalances under control. Eating in a healthy and balanced way can be a cure for PCOS. Yet even our ovarian activity, the epithalamic-pituitary axis that influences all the production of the endocrine glands, and finally the metabolism, are strongly influenced by what we introduce into our body with the daily diet. Other rules to follow, essential to help you dispose of the excess pounds that in PCOS sufferers tend to concentrate dangerously around the waist, are the following:

- **Never skip breakfast:** complete and balanced, with a share of fats and proteins (e.g., a cup of milk without sugar or yogurt), fresh fruit, and complex carbohydrates (wholemeal bread, flakes of cereals or rusks, always whole).

- **Drink lots of water:** It helps the body eliminate toxins, satiates you (sometimes what looks like appetite, is just thirsty), and cleans your skin. Avoid sugary and bubbly drinks, but also pay attention to alcohol and soft drinks, better avoid them. If anything, consume green tea that helps reduce hunger and contains antioxidants, and draining herbal teas.
- **Cooking simply**: steamed, grilled, in a pressure cooker, etc. Avoid elaborate and lengthy cooking, browning, and frying. Do not boil the vegetables in water, because they lose many of their nutritional properties.
- **Eat three full meals a day**: with carbohydrates, proteins, and vegetables, possibly even in a single dish - and two light snacks mid-morning and mid-evening, preferably fruit-based with a low glycemic index (an apple, a cup of berries or strawberries, an orange).

Supplements

Integrating nutrition with specific food supplements is crucial in the case of PCOS. Women who suffer from this syndrome tend to have a deficiency of some critical vitamins and nutrients. Here are some accessories to memorize and on which you can talk to your doctor:

- Inositol
- Vitamin D
- Magnesium
- Omega 3

Risks and complications

In addition to infertility, it is associated with various conditions of metabolic alteration and can also cause serious complications, if underestimated.

- **Diabetes**: It is estimated that over half of women diagnosed with PCOS develop type 2 diabetes before the age of 40, or otherwise come to a pre-diabetes condition.
- **Hypertension**: Too high blood pressure in a young woman is associated with insufficient production of female hormones, which perform a protective function against the cardiovascular system and keep the pressure within limits.
- **Metabolic changes**: again, due to overweight and hormonal imbalance, in women with polycystic ovaries, the values of cholesterol and triglycerides in the blood tend to exceed the guard levels, which, in turn, increases the cardiovascular risk.
- **Night apneas**: In this case, the cause is overweight: since PCOS very often involves weight gain, and even obesity, which in turn is the main cause of obstructive sleep apneas, we can deduce that PCOS is also the first cause of this complication.
- **Mood disorders**: anxiety and depression are a possible consequence of PCOS, and it is a fairly frequent complication, often associated with eating disorders (especially bulimia and compulsive binge eating).
- **Hepatic steatosis and non-acolic steatohepatitis**: these are liver changes that can compromise liver function. The cause is an accumulation of fat, which inflames the liver tissues.
- **Abnormal uterine bleeding** (blood loss between one cycle and another).

- **Endometrial cancer**: irregular cycle and anovulatory cycles, diabetes, overweight, and insulin resistance syndrome, or the whole range of possible complications related to polycystic ovary syndrome contributes to increasing the risk of this type of cancer.

For all these reasons, PCOS should not be underestimated, although discovering that you are part of that 10% of women who suffer from it is an event that should not be dramatized, but addressed. You can get out of it, and there are many resources at your disposal.

Chapter 2: PCOS and diet

Eating in a healthy and balanced way can be a cure for PCOS. Our ovarian activity, the epithalamic-pituitary axis that influences the entire production of the endocrine glands, and finally, the metabolism, are strongly influenced by what we introduce into our body with the daily diet. There are foods, and drinks, which not only help make us fat, but which induce states of sub-inflammation, slow down the liver and pancreatic activity and ultimately increase insulin production.

Foods to eat

- unprocessed natural foods;
- high-fiber foods;
- fat fish, such as salmon, tuna, sardines and mackerel;
- cabbage, spinach and other green leafy vegetables;
- red fruits, such as red grapes, blueberries, blackberries and cherries;
- broccoli and cauliflower
- beans, lentils and other legumes;
- healthy fats, such as those contained in olive oil, avocado and coconuts;
- dried fruit such as pine nuts, walnuts, almonds and pistachios
- dark chocolate in moderation
- spices, such as turmeric and cinnamon

Foods to avoid

- refined carbohydrates, such as sweets and white bread;
- fried foods, fast food;
- sugary drinks, such as carbonated drinks and energy drinks;
- processed meats, such as hot dogs, sausages, frankfurters and prepackaged meat-based foods;
- solid fats, including margarine, butter and lard;
- excess red meat.

Example meal plan

Day 1

Breakfast

Partially skimmed cow's milk 200ml

Corn Flakes Cereals 30g

Snack

Apple 150,0g

Wholemeal rusks 25.0g

Lunch

Spelled soup 60.0g

Grilled turkey breast 100.0g

Aubergines (pan) 150.0g

Extra virgin olive oil 10.0g

Snack

Partially skimmed milk yogurt 125.0g

Wholemeal rusks 25.0g

Almonds 15,0g 86,3kcal

Dinner

Baked sea bass 100.0g

Fennel (raw) 150.0g

Whole wheat bread 75.0g

Extra virgin olive oil 10.0g

Day 2

Breakfast

Partially skimmed cow's milk 200.0ml

Muesli Cereals 30.0g

Snack

150,0g Oranges

Wholemeal rusks 25.0g

Lunch

Barley soup

Pearl barley 60.0g

Grilled chicken breast 100.0g

Zucchini (in a pan) 150.0g

Extra virgin olive oil 10.0g 90.0kcal

Snack

Partially skimmed milk yogurt 125.0g

Whole meal rusks 25.0g

Walnuts, dried 15.0g 99.0kcal

Dinner

Baked fillet of sea bream 100.0g 90.0kcal

Witloof chicory or Belgian endive (raw) 150.0g

Whole wheat bread 75.0g

Extra virgin olive oil 10.0g

Day 3

Breakfast

Partially skimmed cow's milk 200.0ml

Corn Flakes cereals 30,0g

Snack

Kiwi 150,0g

Whole meal rusks 25.0g

Lunch

Beans in broth 70.0g 217.7kcal

Grilled veal loin 100.0g

Pumpkin (baked) 150.0g

Extra virgin olive oil 5,0g

Snack

Partially skimmed milk yogurt 125.0g

Whole meal rusks 25.0g

Hazelnuts 15,0g 94,2kcal

Dinner

Pan-fried cod fillet 100.0g

Chard or chard (boiled) 150.0g

Whole wheat bread 75.0g

Extra virgin olive oil 10.0g

Day 4

Breakfast

Partially skimmed cow's milk 200.0ml

Muesli Cereals 30.0g

Snack

Pink grapefruit 150.0g

Whole meal rusks 25.0g

Lunch

Chickpeas in broth 70g

Shrimp in a pan 100.0g

Cabbage (raw) 150.0g

Extra virgin olive oil 5,0g

Snack

Partially skimmed milk yogurt 125.0g

Whole meal rusks 25.0g

Pine nuts 15,0g 94,4kcal

Dinner

Partially skimmed milk ricotta 100.0g

Potatoes (boiled) 100.0g

Whole wheat bread 75.0g 1

Extra virgin olive oil 5,0g

Day 5

Breakfast

Partially skimmed cow's milk 200.0ml

Corn Flakes cereals 30,0g

Snack

Pears 150,0g

Whole meal rusks 25.0g

Lunch

White risotto 60.0g

Natural tuna, drained 80.0g

Broccoli (boiled) 150.0g

Extra virgin olive oil 5,0g

Snack

Partially skimmed milk yogurt 125.0g

Whole meal rusks 25.0g

Pecan nuts 15,0g

Dinner

Boiled eggs 60.0g

Artichokes (stewed) 150.0g

Whole wheat bread 75.0g

Extra virgin olive oil 5,0g

Day 6

Breakfast

Partially skimmed cow's milk 200 ml

Muesli Cereals 30.0g

Snack

Apple 150,0g

Whole meal rusks 25.0g

Lunch

Spelled soup 60.0g

Grilled pork loin 100.0g

Aubergines (pan) 150.0g

Extra virgin olive oil 5,0g

Snack

Partially skimmed milk yogurt 125.0g

Whole meal rusks 25.0g

Almonds 15.0g

Dinner

Octopus salad 100.0g

Fennel (raw) 150.0g

Whole wheat bread 75.0g

Extra virgin olive oil 10.0g

Day 7

Breakfast

Partially skimmed cow's milk 200.0ml

Corn Flakes cereals 30,0g

Snack

150,0g Oranges

Whole meal rusks 25.0g

Lunch

Barley soup 60.0g

Chicken breast 100.0g

Zucchini (in a pan) 150.0g

Extra virgin olive oil 10.0g

Snack

Partially skimmed milk yogurt 125.0g

Whole meal rusks 25.0g

Walnuts, dried 15.0g

Dinner

Baked monkfish fillet 100.0g

Witloof chicory or Belgian endive (raw) 150.0g

Whole wheat bread 75.0g 182

Extra virgin olive oil 10.0g

Chapter 3: Breakfast

Note: all recipes have been designed for 4 people

1) Potato omelette

Ingredients:
- **Eggs 4**
- **Potatoes 300 g**
- **Parmesan cheese 70 g**
- **Parsley to taste**
- **Salt to taste**
- **Black pepper to taste**
- **Seed oil to taste**

Finely chop the parsley. Peel the potatoes and cut them into 1 cm long slices. Bring a pot full of water to the boil and then blanch the sliced potatoes for 4-5 minutes. Now pour the eggs into a bowl, add the grated cheese, the chopped parsley, and salt and pepper. At this point, mix to mix the ingredients. Drain the potatoes that have finished cooking, let them cool, and then add them to the egg mixture. Take a pan, heat a drizzle of seed oil, and pour the dough once it is hot. Cover with the lid and cook over moderate heat for 15 minutes, turning the pan occasionally. When the surface is not very soft but still damp, turn the omelette over the lid, turning the pan over. Slide the omelette back into the pan to cook the other side, cover again with the lid and continue cooking for another 5 minutes. After this time, the omelette will be ready, and you can serve it hot or cold.

2) Avocado and raspberry toast

Ingredients:

- **6 slices of wholemeal bread**
- **1 avocado**
- **1 lime**
- **50 g of fresh raspberries**
- **salt**
- **balsamic vinegar**

First, clean the avocado. Cut it in half and make some slices, mash the rest with a fork, seasoning it with salt and lime juice. Brush the slices of bread with the oil and toast them a couple of minutes on each side, so that they appear golden brown. Spread the avocado cream on the bread, then add the whole raspberries and avocado slices. Decorate with a few drops of balsamic vinegar: the avocado and raspberry toast is ready!

3) Coconut pancakes

Ingredients:

- **1 eggs**
- **150 ml of coconut milk**
- **90 g of almond flour**
- **250 g of coconut flour**
- **1 teaspoon of baking powder**
- **10 g honey**

Break the eggs in a bowl, add the coconut milk, honey, salt, and mix. Add the flour, coconut flour, and baking powder. Stir until a smooth and homogeneous batter is obtained. Cook the pancakes now by placing a ladle of batter at a time in a lightly buttered pan. As soon as bubbles form on the pancake's surface, turn it over and cook the other side. Gradually stack the pancakes obtained by placing them on top of each other on a flat plate. Serve the pancakes with coconut flakes on the surface.

4)   Japanese omelette

Ingredients:
- **3 eggs**
- **1 tbsp dashi**
- **1 teaspoon of brown sugar**
- **1/2 teaspoon of soy sauce**
- **seed oil**

Mix the dashi, soy sauce, and brown sugar. Pour everything into a bowl in which you will have opened the eggs. Then beat the eggs by mixing the ingredients. Pour 1/5 of the preparation into a pan with a little hot oil. When the crepe is cooked, roll it towards one edge of the pan. Pour 1/5 of the preparation on the opposite side and spread it under the first roll. As soon as this crepe is also cooked, roll it around the ready one. Repeat the operation until you finish the beaten eggs forming an omelette rolls. Leave to cool and cut the roll into slices.

5) Milk biscuits

Ingredients:
- **250 g of almond flour**
- **1 teaspoon of baking powder**
- **1 pinch of salt**
- **1 teaspoon of vanilla essence**
- **150 g of fat-free butter**
- **170 g of skim milk**

Put the flour in a bowl, make a hole in the center and add all the other ingredients. Knead until a soft and homogeneous dough is obtained. Form a homogeneous ball, cover the dough with plastic wrap and let it rest in the fridge for 30 minutes Spread the dough on a floured pastry board, cut out the biscuits with the shape you prefer Put the biscuits on a baking tray covered with parchment paper, brush them with a little milk and bake them in a preheated oven at 200 degrees for about 10 minutes. Allow the milk biscuits to cool before serving.

6) Cookies with wholemeal flour and honey

Ingredients:
- **90 g of honey**
- **45 ml of olive oil**
- **1 egg**
- **250 gr of whole wheat flour**
- **1 teaspoon of baking powder**
- **1 orange peel**

In a bowl, mix the egg with the oil and honey. Add the whole wheat flour, baking powder, and grated orange peel. Work until a soft and homogeneous dough is obtained. With the dough obtained form balls and place them on a baking tray covered with parchment paper. Mash the balls with the prongs of a fork, then bake the biscuits in a preheated oven at 160 degrees for 15 minutes. Leave to cool and serve the biscuits with wholemeal flour and honey.

7)   Muffins with chocolate chips

Ingredients:
- **Fat-free butter softened at room temperature 125 g**
- **Almond flour 265 g**
- **Stevia 135 g**
- **Room temperature skimmed milk 135 g**
- **Eggs (about 2) at room temperature**
- **Dark chocolate drops 100 g**
- **Vanilla bean 1**
- **Satin bicarbonate 1 tsp**
- **Salt up to a pinch**
- **Baking powder for cakes 10 g**

Work the butter with the electric whisk, let it soften at room temperature for at least an hour previously, with the stevia, until a creamy mixture is obtained. Then cut a vanilla bean and scrape the seeds using the back of a knife. Add them to the bowl with butter and sugar. Operate the whisk again and add the eggs one at a time. Now sift the flour, baking powder, and baking soda directly into the bowl with the mixture. Also, add a pinch of salt and operate the whisk again to incorporate the powders. You will notice that the dough will become more consistent, then dilute it with milk at room temperature poured flush. Add 80 grams of chocolate chips and mix them with a spatula to incorporate them. Place the paper cups in a muffin pan and fill them 2/3 full, leaving less than an inch from the surface. Each muffin will have to weigh approximately 70 grams. Pour the remaining chocolate chips over the cupcakes and bake in a preheated oven at 180 ° for 18-20 minutes in static mode. At this point, your chocolate chip muffins are ready to be enjoyed.

8) Sponge cake

Ingredients:
- **Eggs 5**
- **Stevia 150 g**
- **Vanilla bean 1**
- **Gluten-free corn starch 150 g**

Start by placing the eggs (at room temperature) in a planetary mixer, then add the stevia and whisk the ingredients for at least 10/15 minutes with the whisk until you get a frothy, swollen, and light yellow compound. If you wish, when the mixture is well whipped, you can add the vanilla bean seeds that you have cut in half and continue whipping a few seconds to mix it well and flavor the dough. You can add the corn starch that you have previously thoroughly sieved: mix everything with a wooden spoon until a homogeneous mixture is obtained, taking care not to disassemble it. Grease and flour well with corn starch, a round baking pan with a diameter of about 24 cm, pour the dough into the mold's center, leveling it well. Bake the sponge cake gluten-free for about 35-40 minutes at 180 ° C in a preheated oven without ever opening the oven in the first half-hour of cooking. Remove the mold from the oven and let the sponge cake cool in the mold before opening it. Excellent in milk!

9)   Brioche without sugar

Ingredients:
- **250 g Coconut flour**
- **100 g Mother yeast**
- **140 ml Skimmed milk**
- **1 egg**
- **50 g Fat-free butter at room temperature**
- **50 g Coconut Sugar**
- **a pinch of salt**
- **1 yolk (for brushing)**
- **1 teaspoon Coconut Sugar**

Melt the yeast with the milk and sugar. Leave to rest, covered, for 20 minutes. Transfer the mixture to a bowl, preferably planetary, and add the flour. Knead and add the egg until it is completely incorporated. Add a pinch of salt and continue kneading, add a piece of butter at a time, and incorporate it completely before adding the other piece. Let rise, covered with plastic wrap. We can do it in the oven with the light on until doubled, or put in the fridge overnight, where it will rise more slowly but optimally. Once the dough is brought back to room temperature, add a 12 cm pan with the butter and flour it. Pour the dough and level it. Brush the surface with egg and sprinkle with a teaspoon of coconut sugar. Preheat the oven to 200 ° C and bake the brioche for 30 minutes, taking care after ten minutes to lower the power to 170 °. Before turning out of the oven, we do the toothpick test. Remove from the oven and transfer the sugar-free brioche to a wire rack to cool. Delicious with milk for a tasty breakfast!

10) Wholemeal rusks

Ingredients:
- **250 g of whole wheat flour**
- **30 ml of seed oil**
- **1 egg**
- **125 ml of skim milk +5 ml for brushing**
- **2 g of dry brewer's yeast**
- **2 g of salt**
- **two spoons of spoons of honey**

Place the two flours in the bowl of a planetary mixer, if you do not have a planetary mixer, knead with your hands. Add the brewer's yeast to the two flours, mix. Add the honey and milk and start kneading until the powders have completely absorbed the milk. Then add the egg, honey, oil, and salt and knead until a smooth and homogeneous mixture is obtained. Make a sausage. Arrange it in a plum cake pan of about 24X12 cm and let it rise, covered with cling film, for at least 3 hours or until the mixture has tripled in volume. In the meantime, preheat the oven to 180 C. Brush the surface with 10 ml of milk. Bake for about 20 minutes, test the toothpick: it will have to come out clean and dry from the center. Leave the bread to cool completely. Cut it into 20 equal slices. Arrange the slices on a baking tray covered with parchment paper and toast them for 20 minutes in a hot oven, preheated to 150 ° C. When they are golden and crispy, take them out of the oven. Keep them in a tin box or a polypropylene bag for food.

11) Savory herb pancakes

Ingredients:

- **Medium eggs 2**
- **Almond flour 100 g**
- **Skimmed milk 70 ml**
- **Gruyere cheese 50 g**
- **Chopped chives 1 tbsp**
- **Chopped parsley 2 tbsp**
- **Chopped basil 1 tbsp**
- **Instant yeast for savory preparations ½ tsp**
- **Salt to taste**
- **Black pepper to taste**
- **Extra virgin olive oil 2 tbsp**

FOR THE CREAM

- **Sour cream (or very thick Greek yogurt) 80 g**
- **Chopped chives 1 tbsp**
- **Salt to taste**
- **White pepper to taste**

Start grating the gruyere coarsely and set it aside. Chop the chives, basil, and parsley. In a bowl, put the sifted flour and baking powder, add the grated cheese, and chop herbs: parsley, chives, and basil. In a separate bowl, beat the eggs with the milk and add the liquid obtained in the bowl containing the rest of the dry ingredients. Mix well until a soft and homogeneous mixture is obtained. In a small non-stick pan, put 2 tablespoons of extra virgin olive oil and heat it on the fire: take 3 tablespoons of dough at a time and lay them in a pan, forming 3 pancakes that you will cook on both sides until they become golden 12. Remove the pancakes from the pan, drain them on paper towels, and keep them warm; put another spoonful of olive oil in the pan and pour the remaining pancakes in the same way. Prepare the cream that will accompany the salted pancakes by mixing the sour cream (or Greek yogurt) and half a tablespoon of chopped chives, salt, and pepper evenly in a bowl. Serve the savory herb pancakes with a spoonful of cream on each and a sprinkling of leftover chives.

12) Savoury cake

Ingredients:
- **Wholemeal flour 250 g**
- **Light cold butter 125 g**
- **Cold water 85 g**

FOR THE STUFFING
- **Sweet potatoes 200 g**
- **Brussels sprouts 120 g**
- **Red onions ½**
- **50 g bresaola**
- **Basil to taste**
- **Extra virgin olive oil to taste**
- **Salt to taste**
- **Black pepper to taste**

First, put the flour, the butter cut into cubes in the container of a mixer equipped with blades, and blend everything until a sandy mixture is obtained. Then, always with the mixer in action, at moderate speed, add the water flush. As soon as you have obtained a uniform mixture, transfer the dough to a lightly floured surface and knead it for a few moments. At this point, wrap in plastic wrap and let stand for about 30 minutes in the refrigerator. In the meantime, take care of preparing the filling. Wash the sweet potatoes well and, without peeling them, cut them into very thin slices using a mandolin; gradually transfer them to a bowl full of water so as not to oxidize them. Cut the onion into thin slices and transfer it to a pan where you have already poured a drizzle of oil. Let it dry and, in the meantime, take the bresaola and cut it with a knife. Wash and cut the sprouts into thin slices and as soon as the onion has dried, add the bresaola to the pan. Stir until it is well browned, then add the sprouts too. Season with salt, pepper, and cook over medium heat for a few minutes. Preheat the oven to 200 ° C, then butter and flour a 24 cm mold. Take the dough and roll it out with a rolling pin until it is half a cm thick. Then transfer the dough into the mold and press lightly with your fingers to make it stick. With a small knife, remove the excess of pasta from the edges and using a fork, prick the base. Place the first layer of potatoes and add the mixture of bresaola and sprouts. Arrange the potato slices left around only, leaving a space in the center. Add the basil leaves, break them up with your hands and season with salt and pepper. At this point, bake in a preheated oven at 200 °, in the lowest shelf, for about 35 minutes. Then move the pan to the center shelf and cook for another 20 minutes. As soon as the savory pie is cooked and golden brown, take it out of the oven and serve it.

Chapter 4: Snack, Side, Appetizers

1)   Hummus

Ingredients:

- **Pre-cooked chickpeas 500 g**
- **Sesame seeds 800 g**
- **Hot water 120 g**
- **½ lemon juice**
- **Sesame oil 20 g**
- **Paprika 1 tsp**
- **Garlic 1 clove**
- **Salt to taste**
- **Black pepper to taste**
- **Parsley 1 sprig**

Start by chopping the garlic clove and the parsley. Pour the sesame seeds into a pan and toast the seeds over low heat for 2-3 minutes. Then transfer them to a mixer and blend. Add the sesame oil flush, a pinch of salt, hot water, and continue stirring. Then add the drained pre-cooked chickpeas and continue to mix and blend. Squeeze the juice of half a lemon and add the garlic, chopped parsley, salt, and pepper again and mix again. Once the hummus is ready, you can flavor again with fresh parsley, smoked paprika, and a drizzle of seed oil, so your hummus is ready! Serve it as an appetizer with fragrant wholemeal bread bruschetta or for a Middle Eastern-themed dinner with azimo or Arabic bread lightly toasted in the oven!

2)   Potato burger

Ingredients:
- **Potatoes 650 g**
- **Red onions 140 g**
- **Breadcrumbs 60 g**
- **Grana Padano to be grated 50 g**
- **Eggs 1**
- **Water 40 g**
- **Extra virgin olive oil 20 g**
- **Thyme 2 sprigs**
- **Sage 2 sprigs**
- **2 sprigs rosemary**
- **Salt to taste**
- **Black pepper to taste**

FOR THE SALAD
- **Savoy cabbage 80 g**
- **Spinach 40 g**
- **Green apples 80 g**
- **Greek yogurt 100 g**
- **Extra virgin olive oil 10 g**

First, boil the potatoes in boiling water for about 40 minutes or until they are soft. Clean the onions, slice them, heat the olive oil in a saucepan, add the onions, cover them with water, and stew for about 15 minutes until they are soft. Meanwhile, chop the thyme, sage, and rosemary and set aside. In the meantime, prepare the salad: divide the cabbage in half, remove the central hard rib, then reduce it to thin strips. Collect the cabbage in a bowl, salt it, and let it rest for about 30 minutes. Meanwhile, wash and dry the apples, and cut them into thin slices, reduce each slice to strips and keep them aside. Now dry the cabbage with a cloth. In a bowl, pour the washed and dried spinach, add the savoy cabbage, the apples, the yogurt, the olive oil, and mix. When the potatoes are ready, put them in the potato masher, collecting the puree in a large bowl. Also, add the grated cheese, the chopped herbs, salt, and pepper. Also, add the stewed onions, the beaten egg, then add the breadcrumbs one spoonful at a time to obtain a compact mixture; the dough may require more or less than the dose indicated based on the consistency of the compound. Everything is ready to form the burgers: cut out a square of parchment paper about 12 cm on each side and lay it on a saucer. Place a 10 cm diameter round pastry cutter in the center of the sheet, insert the dough inside the pastry cutter, and press it well with the spoon's back. Remove the pastry cutter gently: you will have obtained your burger. Now move on to cooking: heat a pan with a drizzle of olive oil, lay the burger up with the paper so that it remains compact. Once placed on the pan, remove the parchment paper. Cook the burgers 3 minutes on one side and 2 minutes on the other, they must be golden on the surface. Serve the hot potato burgers immediately with the yogurt salad.

3) Eggplant rolls

Ingredients:

- **Long aubergines (4 slices) 120 g**
- **Mozzarella 100 g**
- **Tomato sauce 200 g**
- **Pitted Taggiasca olives 15 g**
- **Basil 4 leaves**
- **Garlic 1 clove**
- **Extra virgin olive oil 2 tbsp**
- **Salt to taste**
- **Black pepper to taste**

Heat the oil in a saucepan, add a clove of garlic and cook it for 5 minutes over low heat. When the oil is flavored, pour the tomato pulp, pepper, salt, and cook for another 15 minutes. In the meantime, wash the aubergine and cut it into slices about 1 cm thick: you will have to make 4 long slices of uniform thickness. Heat a plate well, grill the aubergine slices on both sides, and then transfer them to a plate. When the tomato sauce is ready, remove the garlic clove. Chop the mozzarella and preheat the oven to 180 °. Spread a layer of tomato on the aubergines' surface, add a little frayed mozzarella, a teaspoon of olives, and a basil leaf. Roll up the aubergines and place them in a small baking dish with the closure facing down. Finally, cover the rolls with a little tomato sauce and a few other pieces of mozzarella. Bake them in the oven at 180 ° for about 10 minutes, just long enough to melt the cheese. Once baked, your eggplant rolls are ready to be savored again!

4)   Salmon rolls

Ingredients:
- **160 g of sliced smoked salmon**
- **300 g of light spreadable fresh cheese**
- **1 lime (juice and zest)**
- **1 ripe avocado**
- **fresh dill**
- **salt**
- **pepper**

In a bowl, mix the cheese with the finely chopped dill and the grated lime zest. Season with salt and pepper: you will need to obtain a homogeneous cream that you will transfer for convenience to a sac-à-poche. Divide the avocado in half, remove the peel, and cut it into slices of about 1 cm. Transfer them to a plate and drizzle them with the filtered lime juice. Spread a slice of smoked salmon on the work surface, place a little cream cheese on top and place an avocado stick on top. Roll up to form a roll. Proceed in this way until the ingredients are used up, arranging the rolls on a plate. Finish with a few leaves of dill. Keep the smoked salmon rolls, cream cheese, and dill in the refrigerator until ready to serve.

5) Anchovies marinated in lemon

Ingredients:
- **500 g clean anchovies**
- **30 ml vinegar**
- **4 lemons**
- **1 clove of garlic**
- **2 fresh red chillies**
- **pink pepper**
- **6 sprigs of parsley**
- **salt**
- **extra virgin olive oil**

In a mixer, blend the lemon juice filtered with the parsley, garlic, salt, vinegar, and extra virgin olive oil until a homogeneous emulsion is obtained. In a pan lay the cleaned anchovies with the inside facing upwards and drizzle with the emulsion, the chili pepper, and the pink peppercorns and leave to marinate in the refrigerator for at least 5 hours. Once ready, transfer the marinated anchovies with lemon to a serving plate and garnish with lemon zest and a drizzle of oil. Serve as an appetizer during a fish lunch or dinner.

6) Rice and onion pie

Ingredients:
- **450 g of white onions**

- **320 g of brown rice**
- **4 spoons of olive oil**
- **a knob of butter**
- **salt**
- **pepper**

In a pan, heat a few tablespoons of oil and let the onions cut into very fine slices, season with salt and pepper. Boil the rice in salted water, drain it al dente, season it with a little butter. Arrange a rice layer in a buttered mold, cover it with one of the onions, put more rice on top, and so on until you run out of ingredients. Bake at 180 degrees for twenty minutes. Withdraw, leave the pie for ten minutes and then turn it upside down on a serving plate. Serve.

7) Gratin potatoes

Ingredients:
- **800 g of potatoes**
- **Fat free butter 50 g**
- **grated Parmesan cheese**
- **100 g of sliced raw ham**
- **salt**
- **black pepper**

Start to peel and wash the potatoes well. Cut them into slices about 5-6 mm thick. Blanch them in salted water for 6-8 minutes, then drain them and let them cool. Preheat the oven to 200 C. In the meantime, butter the bottom of an oven dish. Place the first layer of potatoes in slightly overlapping slices and follow with a sprinkling of cheese and ground pepper. Spread the ham cut into thin strips on top. Repeat the layers until the ingredients are use up.

Sprinkle the last with abundant Parmesan cheese and a few walnuts of butter. Bake in the preheated oven at 200 ° for about 40 minutes or until golden brown. Remove from the oven the potatoes au gratin, let them settle for a few minutes and serve.

8) Mussels marinara

Ingredients:
- **2 kg of mussels**
- **1/2 glass of white wine**
- **a bunch of parsley**
- **1 clove of garlic**
- **extra virgin olive oil**
- **black pepper**

To prepare mussels marinara, you must first clean the mussels thoroughly. Remove the broken or empty ones and put the rest in a pot with rather high edges in which you will have put a round of oil. Bring the saucepan over high heat and add the wine, the garlic clove, and the parsley (chopped or whole to taste). Lightly pepper and cover. As soon as the valves open, the mussels are ready. Transfer them to a serving dish and drizzle them with the filtered cooking liquid through cheesecloth. Serve the mussels marinara immediately!

9) Rice Pizza

Ingredients:
- **200 gr of rice**
- **1 egg**
- **1 sachet of saffron**
- **50 g of grated Parmesan**
- **100 g of tomato sauce**
- **100 g of mozzarella**
- **salt**
- **extravirgin olive oil**

Boil the rice in salted boiling water, drain it al dente and add saffron and Parmesan. Preheat the oven to 200 C. Stir and let cool, then add the egg too. Take the rice one handful at a time: create a meatball, mash it in your hands and place it on the baking tray lined with parchment paper, giving it a round shape. Continue with all the rice. Fill each pizza with 1 tablespoon of tomato sauce (previously seasoned with salt and oil), leaving the edges free, then add a few pieces of mozzarella in the center. Bake for about 5 minutes in a preheated convection oven at 200 ° C: the rice pizzas are ready.

10) Californian wrap

Ingredients:
- **4 wholemeal wrap**
- **300 g of chicken**
- **2 avocados**
- **2 spring onion**
- **2 limes**
- **2 tomatoes**
- **2 cucumbers**

In a pan, roast the chicken. In the same pan, heat the wrap on both sides. In the meantime, clean the vegetables and cut them into thin slices. Then start assembling the first wrap: place a wrap on a plate, arrange the chicken in the center, creating a strip from one end to the other, leaving about 1/3 of the wrap free on each side. Add the onion, cucumber, tomato, and avocado over the chicken, then sprinkle a little lime on the filling. Roll the 2 free edges of the wrap over the filling and cut the roll in half. Proceed in the same way with the second wrap. Your Californian wrap is ready, serve it with sauces to taste.

11) Millet meatballs with vegetables and fava bean cream

Ingredients:
- Organic peeled millet 200 g
- Water 550 g
- Extra virgin olive oil 25 g
- Gluten-free breadcrumbs 50 g
- Parsley (to be minced) 5 g
- Turmeric powder 1 pinch
- Salt up to a pinch
- Garlic 1 clove
- Zucchini 100 g
- Carrots 100 g
- Shallot 15 g
- Aubergines 100 g

FOR BREADING AND COOKING
- Gluten-free breadcrumbs 40 g
- Extra virgin olive oil 20 g

FOR THE CREAM OF BEANS
- Broad beans (shelled) 150 g
- Mint 2 leaves
- Extra virgin olive oil 10 g

Rinse the millet well under a stream of cold water and drain it, finely chop the shallot, and dice the carrot. Cut the aubergine and zucchini into cubes as well and put everything aside. Then heat the oil in a pan and add the millet, let it toast for a few minutes, stirring occasionally, then pour in hot water, add the salt and cook for 25 minutes. Once cooked, transfer the millet into a bowl and let it cool completely. In another pan, cook the shallots in a drizzle of oil over low heat, then add the carrots, then the aubergines, and finally the zucchini. Salt all, and cook for 20 minutes, blending with a ladle of hot water or vegetable broth until they become soft. Now dedicate yourself to the preparation of the fava bean cream: shell them one by one, and once you have shelled all of them, blanch them for about 10-15 minutes. Then pour the beans into a container with high edges, add oil, mint, and salt and blend everything with an immersion blender until you get a creamy mixture. Add to the cold millet: the vegetables, the chopped parsley, a crushed clove of garlic, and the turmeric. Finally, add 50 g of gluten-free breadcrumbs to obtain a consistency suitable for working the meatballs. Then model the meatballs by taking about 25 g of the mixture at a time, giving around and slightly flattened shape, then passing each meatball in the breadcrumbs and continuing until you finish the dough. Bake the meatballs in the oven at 180 ° C for 18-20 minutes. Serve your millet patties.

12) Broccoli pie in a jar

Ingredients:
- **400 g of boiled Broccoli**
- **8 slices Whole wheat bread**
- **an egg**
- **50 ml Fresh liquid cream**
- **60 g raw ham**
- **two pinches of pepper**

On the bottom of two 500 ml jars, place two slices of soaked bread, the boiled broccoli florets, and the chopped ham slices. Add another layer of bread, broccoli, prosciutto. Close the jar and hang on. Program the 600-watt microwave, insert the jar, and start for 6 minutes. In the meantime, prepare the other broccoli pie in a jar using the same procedure. Once the jar has rested for at least 15 minutes, you can unhook it, put it in the microwave and start for a couple of minutes at maximum power. The push of the steam will easily open the cap. Serve your jar and enjoy it!

Chapter 5: Meat

1) Chicken Burger

Ingredients:
- **500 g of chicken breast**
- **300 g of chicken leg meat**
- **2 limes**
- **extra virgin olive oil**
- **green pepper**
- **fresh chives**
- **1 clove of garlic**
- **1 tablespoon of corn starch**
- **Salt**

The first step in preparing chicken marinades with lime marinade is to thoroughly clean the meat from bones and residual waste. Then chop it with a knife tip and transfer the ground beef to a large bowl. Peel the garlic and divide it in half, chop the chives and combine them with the meat, together with the grated zest of 1 lime. Squeeze the juice of 1 lime and 1/2 and pour it on the meat, also adding a spoonful of oil, a pinch of salt, and a sprinkling of freshly ground green pepper. Mix very well with a spoon or with your hands and transfer the covered bowl to the refrigerator for 2 hours. After this time, remove from the fridge, remove the garlic and add the corn starch. Mix well to mix it. Form the burgers now. Place some of the mixture inside a circular hamburger shape, 8 or 10 cm in diameter, resting on parchment paper. Fill up to the edge and, with the back of a spoon, give compactness to the mince, gently remove the ring, and in the same way, prepare the rest of the mixture. Heat a non-stick skillet or pan and, when it is hot, lay the hamburgers with the help of parchment paper. Cook over high heat for about ten minutes, taking care to turn them only halfway through cooking. Serve the chicken burgers with very hot lime marinade, accompanied by a lettuce salad and cherry tomatoes.

2) Meatballs with breading of corn flakes

Ingredients:
- **250 g minced beef**
- **2 tablespoons of grated parmesan**
- **1 egg**
- **chopped parsley**
- **nutmeg**
- **salt**
- **pepper**

FOR BREADING
- **50 g of corn flakes**

Preheat the oven to 180 C. Start to collect the minced meat, chopped parsley, nutmeg, egg, salt, pepper, and grated cheese in a bowl. Work the mixture well with your hands. Form the meatballs a little bigger than a walnut and pan them evenly by rolling them into the corn flakes that you have roughly chopped. Bake them in the oven at 180 degrees for about 25 minutes, turning them halfway through cooking. Serve the corn flakes breaded immediately with one of the sauces written in the following chapters.

3) Turkey roll

Ingredients:

- **1 kg turkey breast in a single slice (open as a book)**
- **15 dried tomatoes in oil**
- **150 g of light ricotta**
- **4 fresh basil leaves**
- **40 g of almonds**
- **20 g pine nuts**
- **50 g of grated cheese**
- **extra virgin olive oil**
- **½ glass of dry white wine**
- **rosemary**
- **salt**
- **pepper**

Preheat the oven to 180 C. In the mixer, blend the dried tomatoes, ricotta, dried fruit, basil, and pecorino. If necessary, add a drizzle of oil until a not too homogeneous cream is obtained. Spread it over the surface of the turkey breast open like a book, reaching a couple of centimeters from the edges. Roll it tight, add salt and pepper. Tie firmly with kitchen string. Place the roll inside an oven dish with a couple of spoons of oil and white wine. Add a sprig of rosemary. Bake in the preheated oven at 180 ° for 60 minutes, adding more white wine if the cooking surface tends to dry out too much. Remove from the oven, transfer to the serving dish, cut into not too thin slices.

4)   Escalopes with mushrooms

Ingredients:

- 600 g of porcini mushrooms
- 400 g of veal slices
- 1 clove of garlic
- wholemeal flour
- extra virgin olive oil
- 20 g of fat-free butter
- salt
- pepper
- fresh parsley

To prepare the mushroom escalopes, start cleaning the mushrooms well and separate the stems from the chapels. Cut the first into cubes and the second into slices. Brown the garlic in the oil in a fairly large saucepan and add the mushrooms. Salt them, pepper them and cook them mixing often. Add some chopped parsley and transfer them to a hot dish. Flour the slices of meat and then shake them slightly to eliminate the excess flour. In the same cooking base of the mushrooms, add the butter and let it melt. Add the slices of meat and cook them on a high flame on both sides, until lightly browned. Add the mushrooms, season with salt and pepper, and leave to flavor for a couple of minutes. Add if you still want some chopped parsley then serve the hot scallops with mushrooms.

5) Chicken skewers with lemon and honey

Ingredients:
- **800 g of chicken breast morsels**
- **2 spoons of honey**
- **2 lime leaves**
- **the juice and zest of 2 lemons**
- **1 clove of garlic**
- **100 ml of extra virgin olive oil**
- **salt**
- **pepper in grains**

TO SEAL THE SKEWERS
- **Bay leaves**
- **3-4 lemons**

In a bowl, mix the filtered lemon juice, the zest, the chopped lime leaves, the sliced garlic, the honey, the crushed peppercorns, and the salt. Add the chicken nuggets and stir. Cover them with plastic wrap and marinate for 30 minutes at room temperature. Drain the chicken nuggets from the marinade and skewer them on the metal skewers alternating them with lemon slices and bay leaves. Cook them on the grill, or the cast iron plate, turning them often for 5 minutes or in the oven for about 20 minutes at 180 C or in any case until the chicken is cooked internally. Serve your lemon and honey chicken skewers immediately.

6)   Saffron chicken and grilled vegetables

Ingredients:
- **400 g of chicken breast**
- **1 diced grilled pepper**
- **1 diced grilled zucchini**
- **1 grilled eggplant cut into cubes**
- **1 onion**
- **wholemeal flour**
- **fresh mint**
- **fresh thyme**
- **1 sachet of saffron**
- **extra virgin olive oil**
- **salt**
- **pepper**

To make the saffron chicken nuggets, start cleaning and cutting the onion, reducing it to thin layers. Also, cut the chicken breast into cubes and quickly flour it in a little flour. Heat a little oil in a large pan and let the onion brown. Add the diced grilled vegetables and brown them until they have softened. Then also add the floured chicken breast cubes and brown them on high heat stirring often. Separately dissolve the saffron in a glass of hot water and add to the pan. Mix the meat and vegetables well, add salt and pepper and bring to the boil. Lower the heat and cook by evaporating the excess liquid. Turn off when the chicken is well cooked and the cooking creamy. Add a few leaves of mint and fresh thyme, a round of raw oil, and immediately serve the chicken nuggets with saffron and grilled vegetables.

7) **Duck in orange sauce**

Ingredients:
- **Duck 2.3 kg**
- **Orange juice 50 g**
- **Melted butter without fat 40 g**
- **Black pepper to taste**
- **Salt to taste**
- **Thyme 3 sprigs**
- **Rosemary 1 sprig**
- **Oranges 3 slices**
- **White wine 30 g**
- **Water 20 g**
- **Extra virgin olive oil to taste**

FOR POTATOES
- **Potatoes 450 g**
- **Salt to taste**
- **Black pepper to taste**
- **5 sprigs rosemary**
- **Extra virgin olive oil 35 g**

FOR THE SAUCE
- **Corn starch 15 g**
- **Stevia 60 g**
- **Oranges 1**
- **Water 20 g**

To prepare the orange duck, get a duck already cleaned of the entrails, the fat, and any feathers. Remove any feathers that are still left by burning them with a blowtorch, rinse them well under running water inside and out, and dry them perfectly with a kitchen towel. Help yourself with an elastic twine for food, knotted the wings passing by the shoulders, and passing on the belly also tie the legs. This will serve to keep the shape of the whole duck well cooked. In a large saucepan, heat the oil. Place the duck and brown it over medium heat on one side and the other. Meanwhile, cut the oranges into slices and when the duck is well browned, transfer it to a baking dish with fairly high edges and fill the inside with three slices of orange, thyme, and rosemary. Then brush the duck with 40 g of melted butter, add salt and pepper and pour about 50 g of orange juice, white wine, and 20 g of water on the bottom of the dish. Before transferring it to the oven, cover the duck with an aluminum foil that you will prick with the fork's prongs to facilitate cooking and not burn the surface of your duck. Transfer to a preheated static oven at 200 ° C and cook the duck with a probe until it reaches 70 ° C in the heart, it will take about 1 hour and 10 minutes. Also, prepare the potatoes which will go to the oven separately but at the same temperature as the duck: wash and clean them with a kitchen cloth, then cut them into possibly equal wedges, leaving the skin; season them in a bowl with oil, salt, and pepper. Then transfer them to a dripping pan lined with parchment paper and flavored with rosemary. Put in the oven with the duck (you can place them in the lower cooking shelf of the oven); they will have to cook at the same temperature for about 30 minutes. In the meantime, dedicate yourself to the sauce: take the orange, peel it, squeeze the juice and filter it, it will take 150 g. Then blanch the orange peel for a few moments in boiling water, then drain and cut into very thin strips. Devote yourself to the sauce by melting the stevia together with the water over very low heat: you will need to reach the temperature of 166 ° C by measuring with a kitchen thermometer and then pour the filtered orange juice; mix with a whisk to emulsify everything and add a few tablespoons of the duck cooking base and the corn starch diluted in 20 g of water. Continue to work the sauce with the whisk until it has thickened, then turn off and strain it through a colander, then add the orange peel, finely sliced and set aside. Once the core temperature is reached, take the duck out of the oven, remove the aluminum foil, brush it with the orange sauce and cook it for about 5/10 minutes on the grill to brown it well. Once golden brown, take out your duck and the potatoes that will be cooked, serve the orange duck on a serving dish with the potatoes and use the orange sauce to sprinkle the slices that you will serve to your guests.

8) Veal with tuna sauce in the ancient way

Ingredients:
- **Baby calf 500 g**
- **Garlic 1 clove**
- **Salt up to 5 g**
- **Black pepper to taste**
- **White wine 40 g**
- **Dried milk 150 g**
- **Drained tuna in oil 125 g**
- **Anchovies in oil 20 g**
- **Capers 20 g**
- **Boiled eggs 4**

- **Vegetable broth 40 g**
- **Extra virgin olive oil 40 g**

Take care to tie your piece of veal with kitchen twine. Tie it so that the piece remains completely still. Season the meat with salt and pepper; do it evenly spread the salt on a cutting board, move it, and collect it. At this point, stack a poached clove of garlic on a toothpick, it will be easier to remove it from the cooking base later. Pour 20 g of oil into a pan that can also be used in the oven and let it warm up. Then add the meat and the garlic clove. Brown the walker over medium-high heat, on all sides for 2-3 minutes. At this point, add the tuna fillets, anchovies, and capers 18. Break the tuna fillets lightly, and when it is toasted and golden brown, blend with the white wine. Once the white wine has reduced slightly, pour in the milk without going directly on the meat. Transfer to a preheated oven at 180 C ° for 7-8 minutes, then turn the walker and continue cooking for another 7-8 minutes. Remove from the oven, cover with silver paper, and allow to cool completely at room temperature. In the meantime, take care of preparing the hard-boiled eggs, cooking them for about 9 minutes after boiling. Once cold, peel them and keep them aside. As soon as the meat has cooled, transfer it to a cutting board and remove the clove of garlic from the cooking surface, then pour the bottom into a mixer container and add the sliced hard-boiled eggs. Start blending with an immersion mixer and add again: 20 g of oil, and the broth. Blend everything until a smooth cream is added, adding more broth if it is too thick. Transfer to the refrigerator to cool it down. Take care of the meat by removing the string and slice it thinly using a very sharp knife. Arrange all the slices of meat on a cutting board, fill them with a teaspoon of cream, place it in the center, and place them on a serving plate. The old-fashioned veal with tuna sauce is ready, and you just have to taste it!

9)   Beef fillet in crust

Ingredients:
- **Beef fillet 1 kg**
- **Fat free butter 40 g**
- **Extra virgin olive oil 20 g**
- **Garlic 1 clove**
- **Sage a few leaves**
- **Rosemary a few sprigs**
- **Salt up to 1 tsp**
- **Black pepper 1 tsp**
- **FOR THE CRUST**
- **Pitted black olives 250 g**
- **Shelled pistachios 150 g**
- **Grated cheese 100 g**

Pour the pitted olives on the cutting board together with the pistachios, then with a knife, you get a beat, not too fine. Collect it in a bowl, add the grated photo, and then stir to make everything even and then keep it aside for a moment. In the meantime, clean the red onion, slice it 3-4 mm thick. Now that everything is ready, sprinkle the cutting board, or the tabletop, with salt and pepper, then lay the beef fillet on top. Rotate it by gently massaging the meat; in this way, the spices will penetrate the tissues. Move to the stove and put a pan on the stove, let the butter melt and season with sage, rosemary and a clove of garlic. Also, add the oil, and when the bottom is warm enough, lay the fillet. Let the meat seal, at medium-high temperature, for about 3 minutes on each side. Occasionally wet the surface to keep the meat moist. When the fillet is fully cooked, discard the aromatic herbs and garlic and place the piece of meat on a wire rack with a pan underneath. Pour the batter of olives and pistachios on the surface and handle to make it adhere completely to the meat. Finish cooking in the oven. Bake at 220 ° in a preheated oven for about 12 minutes. As soon as the fillet is cooked, let it cool a few minutes before slicing it and accompany it with one of the sauces chosen from those thoughts in the following chapters. The crusted fillet of beef is ready!

10) Curry chicken with apples

Ingredients:
- **Chicken thighs and thighs 1,5 kg**
- **Fuji apples 500 g**
- **Garlic 1 clove**
- **Copper onions 1**
- **Greek yogurt 150 g**
- **Curry 6 g**
- **Chili powder 2 g**
- **Fresh ginger 30 g**
- **Water 100 g**
- **Extra virgin olive oil to taste**
- **Salt to taste**
- **Black pepper to taste**
- **Parsley to taste**

First, clean the onion and slice it, peel the fresh ginger and mince it. Wash, then cut the apple into irregular pieces of about 2 cm, keeping the peel. Pour a drizzle of oil into a saucepan, add the onion, a clove of garlic and ginger, and sauté over low heat. When the onion is dried enough, turn up the heat and brown the pieces of chicken. Turn the chicken over so that it browns well on all sides and then remove the garlic. Then add the apple pieces and mix everything. Continue cooking and, in the meantime, add the yogurt, chili powder, and curry in a bowl. Stir to mix the sauce. Once the chicken is lightly golden, pour the spice sauce, salt, add the water and cook with the lid on for at least 20 minutes over medium heat. After twenty minutes, remove the lid and continue cooking for another 10/12 minutes. After this time, add the chopped parsley and the chicken curry with apples will be ready, serve it hot!

11) Baked cutlets

Ingredients:
- **500 g sliced chicken breast**
- **q.b. milk**
- **to taste salt**
- **to taste wholemeal or gluten-free breadcrumbs**
- **q.b. origan**
- **q.b. rosemary**
- **to taste extra virgin olive oil**

Take a large bowl, put in the chicken slices and a little milk, the one needed to completely cover the meat. Add a little salt, cover with plastic wrap, and leave the meat to marinate in milk for a good hour, the more you leave it in, the more tender and juicy it is. In a plate, put the breadcrumbs, also add a little chopped oregano and rosemary. Take the chicken slices, remove them from the milk, and pass them in the breadcrumbs on both sides. Put the breaded slices on a plate. Now take a baking sheet, cover it with a sheet of baking paper, and cut out another sheet of baking paper of the same length. Pour a little oil on the baking paper, put the slices on top, add a little oregano and rosemary on each cutlet, finish with a drizzle of oil also on the cutlets. Now cover everything with the other sheet of parchment paper and seal all the edges by folding them. In this way, the meat will not dry when cooked. Cook the cutlets in a preheated oven at 180 ° for about 25 minutes, the slices do not have to be touched during cooking or turned. Once cooked, serve the hot cutlets, you will feel that they are good, they are tender and tasty!

12) Rabbit in cooking pot

Ingredients:
- **450 g Rabbit (pieces)**
- **two tablespoons extra virgin olive oil**
- **10 cherry tomatoes (yellow and red)**
- **a shallot**
- **a cloves of garlic**
- **2 tbsp extra virgin olive oil**
- **2 sage leaves**
- **a bay leaf**
- **a sprigs Rosemary**
- **a tufts Parsley**

- **2 pinches Salt**
- **2 pinches pepper**
- **a spoon White wine**

Clean the rabbit from any fatty parts, wash and dry it. Heat two tablespoons of oil in a pan and brown the rabbit pieces on both sides. In the meantime, wash the herbs, peel garlic and onion and chop everything. Transfer to a glass bowl, season with two tablespoons of oil, stir, and cook in the microwave for two minutes at maximum power. Add the cherry tomatoes to the browned mix, add the rabbit pieces, salt, pepper, and sprinkle with the wine. Mix well and divide everything into two 500 ml jars. Clean the edges of the jars, close and hook. Put a jar in the microwave and cook for 4 minutes at 700 watts. Remove from the oven and let rest, in a closed jar, for at least twenty minutes. In the meantime, cook the other jar. I remind you that the jar becomes like a small pressure cooker. Therefore it should not be opened when hot, and it is during rest that cooking is completed and the vacuum is created. Now your cooking rabbit is ready to be kept in the fridge, where it will keep for about 10 days, or to be served. To open the jar comfortably, just unhook it, put the jar in the microwave and start at the same power used for cooking, for about 3 minutes. The push of the steam will gently open the cap.

Chapter 6: Fish & Seafood

1)   Grilled stuffed squid

Ingredients:
- 4 large whole and clean fresh squids
- 300 g of boiled cannellini beans
- 40 g of grated cheese
- 1 clove of garlic
- 1 glass of white wine
- 1 untreated lemon
- marjoram
- extra virgin olive oil
- salt
- freshly ground black pepper

Start by rinsing the squid under fresh running water and set aside the tufts with the tentacles, which you will roughly chop with a knife. Heat a little oil in a large pan and brown the peeled and crushed garlic clove with the palm of your hand. Add the chopped tentacles and cook over high heat. Also, add the beans, and cook everything for a few minutes. Deglaze with ½ glass of white wine. When the tentacles are golden and cooked, turn off the heat. Remove the garlic and add the cheese. Season with salt and mix. Fill each squid with a mixture of beans, tentacles, and cheese. Close it at the base with a toothpick. Heat the bottom of the grill pan and place the squid without adding oil. Spread a few thin slices of lemon on each squid. Brown a couple of minutes. Drizzle with a drizzle of oil. Turn the squid over, taking care to keep the lemon slices as a base. Deglaze with the remaining wine. Salt lightly. Cook about ten minutes until, by piercing the squid with a toothpick, the fish will not be tender and yielding. Put out the fire. Sprinkle with a little pepper and serve a squid per dish. Remove the toothpick, drizzle with a drizzle of fresh marjoram oil, and a good appetite.

2)   Steamed sea bass

Ingredients:
- **2 sea bass not very large**
- **8 cherry tomatoes**
- **4 small potatoes**
- **2 untreated lemons**
- **1 ginger root**
- **1 clove of garlic**
- **fresh thyme**
- **fresh parsley**
- **extra virgin olive oil**
- **salt**
- **pepper**

To prepare steamed sea bass, remove the entrails, scale, and remove the gills with scissors. In a small bowl, collect the thyme, a little chopped parsley, the garlic cut into slices, the grated peel of ½ lemon, and a grated fresh ginger. Cover everything with a layer of oil and mix. Salt the inside of the belly of each bass and then sprinkle with oil mixed with the aromas using a brush. Place the sea bass in the basket lined with a sheet of wet parchment paper and squeeze them together with the cherry tomatoes cut in half and cover them with the chopped herbs. Cover the surface of each sea bass with one or two thin slices of lemon. Then fill the base pot with water, arrange the peeled potatoes. Place the basket for bunk cooking. Cover and cook about 20 minutes without ever opening. Take the potatoes and arrange them on the serving dishes together with the cherry tomatoes. Put half a sea bass on each plate, drizzle with a round of oil, pepper, and serve.

3) Baked sardines

Ingredients:
- **350 g of sardines**
- **50 g of breadcrumbs**
- **20 g of grated cheese**
- **20 g pine nuts**
- **1/2 clove of garlic**
- **dried oregano**
- **50 g of extra virgin olive oil**
- **salt**
- **pepper**

In a bowl, mix the breadcrumbs, oregano, grated cheese, oil, salt, and pepper. Mix well with a fork, and you will need to obtain a homogeneous mixture. Now dedicate yourself to cleaning fish. Remove the head from the sardines under the jet of running water and slide your thumb along the spine to open them like a book. Remove the bone and wash them by carefully removing the entrails. Preheat the oven to 200 C. Place them in a 20 x 15 cm rectangular pan, just greased with oil, to compose a homogeneous layer. Cover them with a little of the breadcrumbs mixture. Make the second layer of sardines, arranging them in the opposite direction from the first. Cover them with other flavored breadcrumbs and add the pine nuts. Sprinkle with a little oil and cook in the preheated oven at 200 ° for 20 minutes or until golden brown. Remove the sardines in the oven and serve immediately, hot, or after having made them slightly cool.

4)   Fillet of croaker in mango sauce

Ingredients:
- **Fillet of croaker in mango sauce**
- **4 fillets of croaker**
- **2 mangoes**
- **1 carrot**
- **1 zucchini**
- **a handful of confit cherry tomatoes**
- **1 teaspoon granulated sugar**
- **White wine**
- **extra virgin olive oil**
- **licorice powder**
- **salt**
- **pepper**

To prepare the umbrine fillets with mango and licorice sauce, rinse and dry the fish fillets very well. Transfer them to an envelope for vacuum cooking, after sprinkling them with a little salt, and arrange them in an ovenproof dish. Bake in a steam oven at 85 ° for about 10 minutes. In the meantime, peel the mango, cut it into slices, and blend the pulp with a tablespoon of oil, a pinch of salt and ground pepper. Cut the vegetables into slices and cook over low heat in a non-stick pan. Cover and cook for about 5 minutes. After this time, add the sugar and blend with the wine, raising the heat. Continue cooking for another 10 minutes on a low flame. Serve by placing each fillet on a layer of mango sauce. Season with a pinch of ground pepper and complete with glazed vegetables, confit cherry tomatoes, and licorice sprinkling.

5)   Tuna and potatoes meatloaf

Ingredients:

- **500 g of potatoes**
- **320 g of canned tuna in oil**
- **100 g of light spreadable cheese**
- **fresh parsley**
- **2 carrots**
- **10-15 boiled green beans**
- **the peel of 1 untreated lemon**
- **1 teaspoon of pickled capers**
- **1 teaspoon pitted olives**
- **extra virgin olive oil**
- **salt**
- **1 knob of butter without fat**

Boil the potatoes in boiling water for 20 minutes, until completely cooked. In the meantime, clean the carrots, cut them into sticks, and sauté them in a pan with a knob of butter, taking care to keep them crispy and golden. Peel the hot potatoes. With the potato masher, reduce them to a soft pulp in a bowl. Add the drained and crumbled tuna, a little salt, and the spreadable cheese, also drained from the whey. Chop some fresh parsley, add it to the dough and mix well with a fork. Roll out a sheet of aluminum foil, brush it with oil and then place a little of the dough in the center of the sheet: arrange the carrot sticks and the boiled green beans lengthwise. Add more dough and repeat the operation until an oval meatloaf is made. At this point, wrap it in aluminum foil and let it rest in the refrigerator for about two hours. In the meantime, mix the lemon peel, fresh parsley, olives, and well drained capers in a blender. Blend the ingredients. To finish preparing the meatloaf, remove it from the refrigerator, open the aluminum foil, and remove it carefully. Spread the lemon peel mixture over the meatloaf and press until it adheres well. Now you can slice your cold tuna and potato meatloaf and serve it.

6)   Gratin mussels

Ingredients:
- **1 kg of mussels**
- **About 150 g of breadcrumbs**
- **1 cloves of garlic**
- **2 spoons of chopped parsley**
- **20 g of capers**
- **1 dl of extra virgin olive oil**
- **salt**
- **pepper**

To prepare the mussels au gratin, you must first clean them very well. If you have already cleaned them, proceed with the recipe. Put them in a large saucepan and let them open, covered, over a high flame. Drain them immediately and collect the cooking water in a bowl, filtering it through a dense mesh strainer. Remove the empty half shells and arrange those with the valve on the oven tray covered with the appropriate paper. Combine the breadcrumbs with the parsley, garlic, and chopped capers in a bowl. Salt, pepper, and add the oil. Mix well, then add a little of the cooking liquid to obtain a soft mixture (be careful, however, that it does not become too moist and wet). With the help of a teaspoon

spread the mixture on each mollusk, covering it well.
Transfer to a preheated oven at 190 C ° and cook for 5
minutes. Remove the mussels from the oven and serve
them hot or warm.

7)   Baked grouper

Ingredients:
- **4 grouper fillets of 200 g each**
- **1/2 lemon**
- **1 glass of dry white wine**
- **1 red chilli pepper**
- **10 g of salted capers**
- **extra virgin olive oil**
- **salt**
- **pepper**

Preheat the oven to 180 C. Wash and dry the fillets well,
salt, and pepper them in moderation on both sides. Place
them in an oil-coated oven dish by placing them side by
side. Season with a drizzle of oil, sprinkle with white wine
and lemon juice filtered through a strainer. Transfer the
dish to the oven and cook the fish for 15 minutes. After
this time, remove the container and add the well desalted
capers and the crumbled chili pepper to the fish.
Continue cooking for 15 minutes, no more; otherwise, the
fish risks becoming fibrous, occasionally wetting the fillets
with their sauce. Remove from the oven, transfer the
fillets to the serving dishes, drizzle them with the cooking
sauce, and immediately serve the grouper in the oven
prepared in this way.

8)   Salmon fillet with quinoa salad

Ingredients:
- **4 fresh salmon fillets with skin of 150/200 g each**
- **150 g of quinoa**
- **40 g of pecans**
- **1 handful of dried cranberries**
- **200 g of valerian**
- **extra virgin olive oil**
- **raspberry vinegar**
- **salt**
- **pepper**

To prepare the salmon fillet with quinoa salad, wash the quinoa several times, then transfer it to a saucepan. Cover it with plenty of water (about 400 ml) and add a little salt to a boil. Leave to cook for about 15 minutes or at least for the time indicated on the package. Drain well and transfer to a bowl. Let it cool down. Add the chopped walnuts, valerian, dried cranberries, and season with a drizzle of oil and raspberry vinegar. Season with salt and pepper and mix. Cook the salmon in a very hot non-stick pan, just greased with oil. Start on the side of the skin for about 2 minutes, turn and cook for 4 minutes (however, adjust according to the thickness of the fillets). The salmon must be very soft and juicy on the inside. Transfer the fillets to their respective serving dishes. You can complete the dish with one of the sauces written in the following chapters!

9)   Baked squid rings

Ingredients:
- **Medium squid already cleaned 600 g**
- **Breadcrumbs 200 g**
- **Sweet paprika 20 g**
- **Extra virgin olive oil 2 tbsp**
- **Salt to taste**

Cut the mantle into rings one centimeter thick and add these to the tentacles, also cut into small pieces. Now take care of the breading: put the breadcrumbs in a bowl and add the sweet paprika and a teaspoon of salt. Pour the mixture obtained in a large pan, arrange the squid rings and the tentacles, mix them so that the breadcrumbs adhere to all sides. Then pass the squid in a large mesh sieve, place a container under the sieve and shake the sieve to remove the excess breading. Grease a pan with oil, then line it with parchment paper, pressing lightly with your hands to better the paper adheres. Transfer the rings and tentacles of the breaded squid to the pan. Pour the oil and bake in a preheated static oven for 25 minutes at 180 ° C. Once cooked, your baked squid rings will be ready to be brought to the table and enjoyed hot.

10) Sesame tuna

Ingredients:
- **Tuna (4 fillets)**
- **Black sesame seeds 10 g**
- **White sesame seeds 20 g**
- **Artichokes 4**
- **Lemon juice 1**

For the sauce
- **Extra virgin olive oil 35 g**
- **Lemon juice 35 g**
- **Salt to taste**
- **Black pepper to taste**

Start cleaning the artichokes. Then prepare a bowl with cold water and squeeze the juice of a lemon inside: the acidified solution will prevent the clean artichokes from turning black. Cut the part of the stem with the knife, leaving a couple of centimeters from the leaves, peel the artichokes keeping only the most tender heart, and cut off the tip of the leaves that has the thorns. With a paring knife, remove the most superficial layer of the remaining stalk, which is the most fibrous part, divide the artichokes in half and extract the inner beard. As you clean the artichokes, soak them in the acidulated water that you have prepared with the lemon juice. Now prepare the sauce. Squeeze the lemon juice, filter it through a colander, add the olive oil, and emulsify it with a whisk. Salt, pepper, and set aside. Now cut the artichokes into julienne strips, collect them in a bowl and season with half the sauce, the remaining part will be used to season the tuna. In a plate pour the white sesame seeds and the black sesame seeds, mix them. Pass the tuna slices on the seeds to bread them on both sides as evenly as possible. Heat a non-stick pan and only when it is hot, lay the tuna fillets in breadcrumbs and cook over high heat for 1 minute, then turn them over, continue cooking for another minute. So seared the tuna will be raw inside, but if you like, you can extend the cooking according to your taste. Once cooked, transfer the fillets to a cutting board, cut them into slices, and serve immediately garnishing the sesame tuna with the remaining sauce and accompanying it with the artichoke salad.

11) Fish burger

Ingredients:
- **Cod fillet already cleaned 600 g**
- **Grated lemon zest 1 tbsp**
- **Thyme 1 tbsp**
- **Parsley to mince 1 tbsp**
- **Salt to taste**
- **Black pepper to taste**

FOR BREADING
- **Eggs 2**
- **Almond flour to taste**
- **Breadcrumbs to taste**
- **Salt to taste**
- **Black pepper to taste**

Cut the fillets into chunks, place them in the mixer, and chop the cod until you get a homogeneous mince.

Transfer the mixture to a bowl and season with pepper, salt, chopped parsley, thyme, and grated lemon zest, mix well with a fork. Place a sheet of parchment paper on a cutting board and start creating the fish burger. With a spoon, distribute the cod mixture inside an 11 cm diameter pasta dish and press it with the back of the spoon so that the mixture assumes the shape of the pasta dish. Remove the pastry cutter and cut the parchment paper around the burgers; thus, you will be facilitated in lifting them without the risk of flaking them. Preheat the oven to 180 C. Now take care of the breading: beat the eggs with salt and pepper. Begin to bread the fish burgers bypassing them first in the flour then in the eggs and lastly in the breadcrumbs. Place the fish burgers in the oven at 180 ° C for 25-30 minutes. Once cooked, drain the burgers and place them on paper towels to absorb excess oil. Your fish burgers are ready to be brought to the table hot!

12) Orange mackerel

Ingredients:
- **Mackerel 4 whole already cleaned**
- **Orange peel 1**
- **Extra virgin olive oil to taste**
- **FOR MARINATING**
- **Orange juice 2**
- **Extra virgin olive oil 60 g**
- **4 sprigs dill**
- **Garlic 3 cloves**
- **Black pepper in grains 1 tbsp**
- **Salt up to 1 tbsp**

Take care of the ingredients for the marinade: with the back of the spoon, crush the peppercorns, so they release their aroma better and squeeze the juice from the oranges. Peel and slice the garlic thinly. Grease an oven dish with oil, lay the mackerel on top, and season them with another drizzle of oil, the peppercorns, salt, flavored with dill sprigs, and flavored slices of garlic. Finally, sprinkle the fish with half the orange juice, cover with cling film, and leave to marinate for 2 hours in the refrigerator. After the marinating time, pass to cooking: heat a pan with a drizzle of olive oil and, when it is hot, lay the fillets. Leave them to cook over high heat for 4 minutes without touching them, then turn them, sprinkle them with the remaining orange juice and continue cooking for another 2 minutes. Once the sauce has thickened, and the mackerel is well-flavored, they serve immediately, garnishing them with grated orange zest on the surface.

Chapter 7 : Soup & Salad

1) Chickpea soup

Ingredients:
- **Dried chickpeas 300 g**
- **Carrots 1**
- **Celery 1 rib**
- **½ white onions**
- **Leeks 1**
- **Extra virgin olive oil 3 tbsp**
- **2 sprigs rosemary**
- **Salt to taste**
- **Black pepper to taste**
- **Laurel 2 leaves**
- **Vegetable broth 1,5 l**
- **Tomato sauce 60 g**

Begin by soaking the chickpeas. Pour them into a large bowl, cover with water and leave for at least 12 hours. After the time, put a pot with the vegetable broth on the fire to heat it. Meanwhile, drain and rinse the chickpeas. Before cooking, clean the leek: remove the two ends, then cut into thin slices. Then clean the celery and mince it. Continue cleaning and mincing the carrot and onion. Pour the oil into a saucepan, let it a warm-up, and then add the chopped celery, leek, carrot, and onion. To help the vegetable stew better, add a ladle of hot broth, and continue cooking for about ten minutes. At this point, pour the chickpeas, letting them brown for a few minutes. Then add the bay leaf and rosemary. Cover the chickpeas with the hot vegetable stock and finally add the

tomato puree. Stir and cover with the lid. Let cook over
low heat for about 2 hours, adding broth as needed. At
the end of cooking, remove the sprig of rosemary and bay
leaf and season with salt and pepper before serving. Your
chickpea soup is ready!

2) Pumpkin cream

Ingredients:

- **Pumpkin 1 kg**
- **Potatoes 200 g**
- **Vegetable broth 1 l**
- **White onions 80 g**
- **Black pepper 1 pinch**
- **Salt 1 pinch**
- **Extra virgin olive oil 60 g**
- **Cinnamon powder 1 pinch**
- **Nutmeg 1 pinch**

To prepare the pumpkin cream, start by preparing the vegetable broth. Then move on to cleaning the pumpkin, then cut it into cubes. Peel the potatoes and cut them into cubes too. Clean the onion, finely chop it, then transfer it to a pan with the oil and let it pass over low heat. Once the onion has dried, add the pumpkin and potatoes. Also, add a part of the broth to cover all the vegetables. Season with salt and pepper. Leave to cook on low heat for 25-30 minutes, adding more broth from time to time. Once the vegetables are cooked, turn off the heat and blend everything with an immersion blender, until obtaining a smooth and homogeneous cream. Then add the cinnamon nutmeg and mix everything. Your pumpkin cream is now ready!

3)   Cream of leek soup with savory croutons

Ingredients:
- **Leeks 600 g**
- **Potatoes (yellow) 300 g**
- **Vegetable broth 500 g**
- **Extra virgin olive oil 60 g**
- **Black pepper to taste**
- **Thyme 3 sprigs**

FOR CROUTONS
- **Whole wheat bread 100 g**
- **Rosemary to taste**
- **Wild fennel to taste**
- **Oregano to taste**
- **Thyme to taste**

Start cleaning the leek and cut it into slices. Then peel the potatoes, cut them into cubes, and then pour the leek into a pan with the slightly heated oil and brown it over medium heat, stirring with a wooden spoon from time to time. When it is wilted, pour the diced potatoes. Pour the vegetable stock, flavored with pepper and thyme, and cook everything for about 30-35 minutes. When the potatoes are softened, and the leek is cooked, immerse the immersion blender and blend until a homogeneous cream is obtained. Pass the cream in a strainer to make it smoother, and then keep it aside in the heat and dedicate yourself to the croutons. Pour the needles of rosemary, fennel, oregano, and thyme into a blender; then chop everything to obtain a mix of herbs and spices. Slice the bread, cut it into cubes, and place it in a bowl. Season with a spoonful of oil and the mix of chopped herbs and spices. Pour the diced bread into a pan and toast them over high heat. When the croutons are ready too, serve the leek cream and garnish each dish with the savory croutons, the rosemary needles, and serve the leek cream very hot!

4) Vegetable soup

Ingredients:
- **Carrots 40 g**
- **Red onions 40 g**
- **White zucchini 75 g**
- **Salt to taste**
- **Black pepper to taste**
- **Celery 30 g**
- **Auburn tomatoes 175 g**
- **Black beans 100 g**
- **Clean pumpkin 125 g**
- **Extra virgin olive oil 25 g**
- **Leeks 75 g**
- **Clean cauliflower 150 g**
- **Peas 100 g**
- **1 sprig rosemary**
- **Laurel 1 leaves**
- **Water to taste**

To prepare the vegetable soup, start by washing and drying the vegetables. Then take the pumpkin, remove the seeds and internal filaments, and cut it into slices of equal thickness and then into cubes of about 1 cm each side. Wash and peel the zucchini and cut them into cubes.

Then shell the beans, then take the cauliflower, cut it in half and obtain the florets; then, cut the leek from the outside, then cut it into thin slices. Proceed with the tomatoes: remove the stalk and also cut the tomatoes into cubes. Finely chop the onion. Peel and peel the carrots, then chop them with a knife. Finely chop the celery too. To finish, tie the rosemary's sprigs with bay leaves with a string to create an aromatic bunch. Pour the oil, celery, carrots, leek, and onion into a large pot with a lid and sauté gently for about ten minutes, stirring frequently. Once the sautéed vegetables are softened, add the fragrant bunch, and pour the beans. Cover with water: he will have to cover the vegetables with a finger. Wait for the boil to set and cook for 2 minutes. Add the pumpkin and repeat the same procedure: add water until it covers a finger, wait for the boil to resume, and cook for 2 minutes. Then add the cauliflower. Cover with more water, put the lid on, and cook for 25 minutes after boiling again. After 25 minutes, add peas, zucchini, and tomatoes, add water if necessary, season with salt and pepper, and cook again 2-3 minutes after boiling again. Remove the sweet sprig!. The soup is ready!

5)

6) Lentil cream

Ingredients:
- **Dried lentils 250 g**
- **Carrots 1**
- **Celery 1 rib**
- **Shallot 1**
- **Turmeric powder 1 tsp**
- **Extra virgin olive oil to taste**
- **Water 1.5 l**
- **Salt to taste**
- **Black pepper to taste**

First, rinse the lentils well under running water. Then clean the odors, then celery, carrot, and shallot, and chop them with a knife coarsely. Put oil in a pan and add the mince, leaving to flavor over medium heat for 4-5 minutes, stirring occasionally. Then add the turmeric powder, the lentils and mix for 1 minute to flavor everything; finally, cover with cold water. Close with the lid and let it cook for about an hour. After the time, add salt and pepper, blend with an immersion mixer and cook over medium heat for another 40 minutes, to thicken everything. As soon as everything is ready, all you have to do is serve! You can garnish with wholemeal bread croutons.

7)   Winter salad

Ingredients:
- **1 head of late radicchio**
- **2 celery sticks**
- **1 fennel**
- **1 steamed red turnip**
- **2 oranges**
- **extra virgin olive oil**
- **sliced almonds**
- **pink Himalayan salt**

Start cutting the radicchio into small pieces and place it on a large plate. Browse the fennel, removing the hardest external part and slice it thinly, spreading it over the radicchio. Peel the celery stalks and cut them into pieces. Cut an orange, peel it and add it to the vegetables. Toast the sliced almonds and squeeze the second orange, filtering the juice. Prepare dressing by adding a pinch of pink salt, a pinch of pepper, and the oil to the orange juice. Mix well and taste the emulsion to dose the quantities of the various ingredients harmoniously. Cut the beetroot into cubes, add it to the salad only at the last and season with the orange emulsion. Complete with toasted almonds and serve the winter salad immediately.

8)   Cauliflower and cod salad

Ingredients:
- **1 small cauliflower**
- **150 g of olives**
- **150 g of green olives**
- **200 g of peppers in oil**
- **50 g of capers**
- **200 g of pickled onions**
- **1 fillet of cod soaked and desalted (about 300 g)**
- **extra virgin olive oil**
- **a spoonful of vinegar**
- **salt**
- **black pepper**

Clean the cauliflower and reduce it into florets that you will wash under the flow of running water. Cook them in boiling salted water until they are tender. Drain them and set aside. Delicate and peel the cod. Cook it in boiling water until it appears tender. Drain and set aside. Cut the well-drained flakes of pepper into strips and collect them in a large bowl with the green and black olives, capers, and onions, all well drained. Add the cauliflower, a drizzle of oil and a pinch of pepper. Jumbled up. Then add the cod, flaking it with your hands. Mix with the vinegar and correct it if necessary with salt. Let the salad rest for at least 6 hours before serving it, so that the flavors are perfectly mixed.

9) Tasty chicken salad

Ingredients:
- **400 g of boiled or cold roasted chicken**
- **100 g of white celery**
- **lettuce**
- **pitted black olives**
- **capers (optional)**
- **guacamole**
- **salt**
- **black pepper**

Boil the chicken in a pan with boiling water or, if you prefer, roast it in a pan without oil. Once you have made one of the two steps, chop the meat with a knife: the pieces and the frays obtained do not necessarily have to be all of the same sizes. Wash and dry the celery, remove any filaments and then cut it into small pieces. Wash and dry the lettuce leaves. Collect the chopped chicken and celery in a large salad bowl. Cut the lettuce into strips and add it to the chicken with the celery. Prepare the guacamole (the recipe can be found in the following chapters), and distribute it on the salad. Add the black olives, the capers, mix well and season with salt and freshly ground pepper. Serve your chicken salad immediately or keep in the fridge until ready for consumption.

10) Cod salad with polenta chips

Ingredients:

- **2 fillets of cod, already boiled**
- **80 g of cornmeal for polenta**
- **500 ml of water**
- **sage**
- **rosemary**
- **3-4 cloves of garlic**
- **red and yellow cherry tomatoes**
- **Cherry Tomato Confit**
- **salted capers**
- **dill**
- **marjoram**
- **extra virgin olive oil**
- **black pepper**

Preheat the oven to 180 C. Start preparing the cod salad recipe with polenta chips and cooking the polenta. Bring the water to a boil and pour in the cornmeal sprinkle, stirring with a whisk. Cook the polenta at medium-high temperature for the time indicated on the package, about 20 minutes, stirring often. Arrange the cod, cut into slices, in a baking dish, and drizzle it with a little oil. Add the garlic cloves, the chopped sage, and the rosemary needles. Bake it in the oven at 180 ° C for 20 minutes. Spread the polenta on a dripping pan lined with parchment paper, place in the oven 100 ° for 30 minutes, or at least the time necessary to make it crispy. Remove from the oven, let it cool down, remove it from the paper and break it irregularly, thus obtaining some chips. Arrange the dish by transferring the cod, warm and reduced to small pieces, in a bowl. Add the cherry tomatoes, capers, dill, and some marjoram leaves. Season with oil and pepper to taste and serve the cod salad with polenta chips immediately.

11) Cream of white beans and clams

Ingredients:
- **400 gr of already cooked white beans**
- **350 gr of clams**
- **1 clove of garlic**
- **extravirgin olive oil**
- **fresh basil**
- **salt**
- **pepper**

First, clean the clams. Prepare a mixture of garlic and oil, add the clams, close with the lid and cook over medium heat for a few minutes, until they open. Drain filtering the cooking water and set them aside, then shell the clams holding some with a shell to decorate the dish at the end. Put the beans in a bowl with salt, pepper, oil, and a little of the clams' cooking base, then start blending with an immersion blender, adding more cooking water if needed to achieve the consistency you prefer. Pour the cream onto a plate and add the shelled clams. The cream of cannellini beans and clams is ready: decorate with some shells, a little basil, and a couple of croutons and serve hot, warm, or cold.

12) Cream of leeks and potatoes

Ingredients:
- **Leeks 800 g**
- **Potatoes 800 g**
- **Vegetable broth 1 l**
- **Extra virgin olive oil to taste**

- **Salt up to a pinch**

Peel and divide the potatoes in half, then into strips, and finally into small cubes. Peel the leeks, removing the ends, and cut them into slices. Then heat a drizzle of oil in a large saucepan and fry the leeks. Deglaze with a ladle of vegetable broth. Let the vegetable broth evaporate, then add the diced potatoes, mix, salt and pepper to taste. Cover with the remaining broth, cover with a lid and cook for 30 minutes until the potatoes have softened. After this time, transfer everything to a bowl. Pass the mixture with an immersion blender until you get a creamy consistency. If the cream is too thick, add a ladle of vegetable broth. Serve!

13) Russian salad in cooking pot

Ingredients:
- **2 medium potatoes**
- **3 carrots**
- **250 g Frozen peas**
- **salt**

To garnish
- **4 tablespoons fat-free mayonnaise**
- **180 g Tuna in oil**
- **1 tablespoon white wine vinegar**
- **1 tablespoon extra virgin olive oil**

Peel and wash the potatoes and carrots, cut them into regular cubes, and transfer them to a bowl. Add the peas still frozen to the vegetables and a pinch of salt. Mix the vegetables and divide them into two liter jars. Clean the edges of the jars, close with a cap, seal, and hooks. Program the microwave at 750 watts, insert a jar, and start cooking for 8 minutes. At the end of the cooking, leave the closed jar to rest for 20 minutes. During the rest, the vacuum will form, and the cooking will be completed. While the pot rests, cook the other pot of vegetables for Russian salad. Now your base for Russian salad cooked in a jar is ready. It can be stored in the fridge, where it will be kept for a week. When serving, pull the garnish, pour the vegetables into a bowl and season with the oil and vinegar, mix well, and rest for 5 minutes. Then season them with mayonnaise and drained tuna, mixing gently and until everything is well mixed.

Chapter 8: Dessert

1) Brownies cake without sugar

Ingredients:
- **195 grams of almond flour**
- **110 grams 85% dark chocolate**
- **60 grams fat-free butter**
- **80 grams stevia**
- **3 eggs**
- **20 grams bitter cocoa**
- **1 pinch of salt**
- **1/4 teaspoon baking soda**

The first thing to do is to melt the dark chocolate, and this can be done both in a water bath and in the microwave, the important thing is not to burn it. Then add the butter to the melted chocolate, constantly stirring so that it melts quickly. When the butter has completely incorporated, add 80 g of stevia and then the eggs, one at a time, mixing each ingredient well after each addition and mixing. Once this is done, combine the bitter cocoa, the pinch of salt, the baking soda, and the previously sieved flour to avoid lumps. Stir carefully to mix all the ingredients well. At this point, pour the mixture into a pan with high edges and bake in a preheated oven for 40 minutes at about 180 ° C. When it is cooked, you can take out the brownies cake without sugar and remove it from the pan as soon as possible. You can leave it whole or cut it into squares ready to be enjoyed.

2) Almond and pear cake

Ingredients:

- **300 grams pears**
- **2 tablespoon raw brown sugar**
- **120 grams dried figs**
- **200 ml rice milk**
- **100 grams almond powder**
- **100 grams of oatmeal**
- **60 grams chickpea flour**
- **30 grams corn starch**
- **1/2 lemon**
- **1/2 teaspoon baking soda**
- **1/2 teaspoon baking powder**
- **2 tablespoon agave or maple syrup**
- **2 tablespoon seed oil**
- **2 spoonful of flaked almonds**
- **Salt to taste**

Caramelize the pears, diced, with 2 tablespoons of sugar for 4-5 minutes. Drain while keeping the cooking liquid. Cut the figs into small pieces, blend them in the mixer with 100 rice milk, 2 tablespoons of pear liquid, and seed oil until a smooth cream is obtained and set aside. In another bowl, mix the powdered almonds with the flour, starch, and grated zest of the lemon, add juice, the remaining milk, and the syrup. Add the fig cream to the mixture and work to obtain a soft and homogeneous mixture. Add the baking soda, baking powder, and a pinch of salt, mix and add the cooked pears to the mixture. Cover a 22 cm diameter round baking tray with parchment paper, pour the dough, level the surface, sprinkle with flaked almonds and bake at 180 ° for 50 minutes, covering the surface with aluminum foil if the cake darkens too much. Serve the cake cold.

3) Cherries crumble

Ingredients:
- **45 grams of coconut flour**
- **30 grams of almond flour**
- **45 grams fat-free butter**
- **Salt to taste**
- **30 grams brown sugar**
- **30 grams ginger**
- **600 grams pitted cherries**

Mix the coconut flour with the almond flour in a bowl, add the sugar and a pinch of salt, then add the very cold butter (just removed from the refrigerator) cut into cubes of roughly the same size. Quickly knead the ingredients until you get a homogeneous dough; then shell it with your hands, distribute the crumbs obtained on a tray. Transfer the mixture to the refrigerator and let it rest for 12 hours. Prepare the filling: wash the cherries, dry them, remove the stalk, cut them into 4 wedges, remove the core, and collect them in a bowl. In doing this, you should use a pair of disposable latex gloves so as not to stain your hands with the juice of the cherries. Add brown sugar, fresh peeled and grated fresh ginger. Stir to mix everything well, cover the bowl of cherry crumble with cling film and leave to marinate at room temperature for 12 hours. After the indicated time, distribute the marinated cherries with their sauce in 4 bowls with a diameter of about 9 cm. Sprinkle the cherry crumble in equal parts over the cherries, try to cover them entirely, and bake at 180 degrees for 20-25 minutes or until the surface becomes golden. Remove the bowls from the oven, let the crumble cool and then serve it garnished, if you like, with fresh cherries.

4) Flour free chocolate cake

Ingredients:
- **Dark chocolate 85% 340 g**
- **Stevia 200 g**
- **Fat-free butter 170 g**
- **Bitter cocoa powder 150 g**
- **Medium eggs 3**
- **Vanilla extract 5 g**
- **Salt up to 3 g**

First, melt the dark chocolate in the microwave or a bain-marie, and let it cool. In a bowl of a planetary mixer, equipped with a whisk, mix the softened butter at room temperature with the stevia, to obtain a creamy mixture. You can also whip the butter with the whisk of an electric mixer. Add one egg at a time, waiting for the previous one to be well incorporated. Add the vanilla extract; Separately sift the cocoa and add it to the butter, egg and sugar mixture, one spoon at a time. Add the salt and finally, the warm chocolate. Mix all the ingredients with a spatula. Grease and line, with parchment paper, a cake tin with a diameter of 22-24 cm, pour the dough into it, level it with the back of a spoon, and distribute it evenly in the cake tin. Bake the cake in the oven at 180 ° for 30-35 minutes; when a crunchy crust is created, take them out of the oven and cool. And your flourless chocolate cake is ready.

5)   Peaches cheesecake

Ingredients:
- **Gluten-free dry biscuits 200 g**
- **Soybean butter 75 g**

FOR THE CREAM
- **Fresh lactose-free spreadable cheese 525 g**
- **Fresh cream without lactose 250 g**
- **Fructose 160 g**
- **Jelly in sheets 10 g**

FOR DECORATION
- **Nectarines 200 g**
- **Strawberries 60 g**
- **Currant 30 g**
- **Mint to taste**

Start with the biscuit base. Grease a 22 cm hinged mold and line it with parchment paper both at the base and on edge. Pour the gluten-free biscuits into a mixer and blend them until a sandy mixture is obtained. Transfer it to a bowl, then melt the butter and pour it over the biscuit powder. Stir with a spoon and pour everything on the pan's bottom, leveling well with the back of a spoon to cover the whole surface evenly. Leave the base to compact in the fridge for about 30 minutes. In the meantime, prepare the cream: soak the gelatine leaves in cold water for about 10 minutes. At the same time, whip 200 g of lactose-free cream with a mixer with a whisk or an electric mixer. In a separate bowl, pour the lactose-free cream cheese, add the fructose, and work it with an electric mixer until you get a homogeneous cream. Heat the remaining 50 g of cream in a saucepan and melt the well-squeezed gelatin over heat, stirring with a whisk. Let the cream cool with the gelatin and insert it, little by little, into the cream cheese continuing to mix. Add the previously whipped cream to the mixture, mixing with a spatula and practicing movements from the bottom upwards; pour the cream obtained on the biscuit base. Level well with a spatula until a smooth and regular surface is obtained; cover the cake pan with plastic wrap and let the cheesecake harden in the fridge for about 6 hours. At the moment of decoration, wash and cut the peaches into very thin slices, without peeling them. Squeeze the lemon juice and pour it over the peaches to not oxidize them. Remove the cheesecake from the fridge and gently remove the hinge and the edge of parchment paper. Then, with the help of a flat spatula, lift it very gently from the pan and transfer it to a splash or on a plate. Decorate it with peach slices, starting from the outer edge. Make a complete circle with the peaches, then cut the strawberries into slices and draw a second inner circle with them. Wash and dry the currants and complete the decoration in the center of the cake by adding mint leaves. Cut into slices and serve very cold!

6)   Gluten free cream puffs

Ingredients:
- **Gluten-free rice flour 45 g**
- **Lupine flour 30 g**
- **Corn starch (cornstarch) gluten free 30 g**

- **Room temperature eggs (approx. 2)**
- **Yolks (about 1 medium)**
- **Water 150 g**
- **Butter 40 g**
- **Salt up to a pinch**
- **TO SEAL**
- **70% melted dark chocolate 50 g**

Melt the dark chocolate in the microwave or soak in the sea. Pour the water, butter, and a pinch of salt into a saucepan. Bring everything to a boil, then remove from the heat and pour the rice flour. Also, add the cornstarch and lupine flour. Mix well with a wooden spoon until all the ingredients are mixed. Return to the heat and, constantly stirring, cook the mixture for about 1 minute. Transfer it to the bowl of a planetary mixer equipped with a leaf and operate the machine. Pour an egg and wait for it to be well absorbed and then add the second one. When this is well absorbed, add the yolk. Continue to work until an elastic and soft dough is obtained, then transfer it to a sac-à-poche with a 10 mm smooth nozzle. Form the cream puffs on a dripping pan lined with parchment paper; you will have to make 3-4 cm tufts, spacing them apart. Bake at 200 ° C for about 25-30 minutes. Then take out the gluten-free cream puffs, let them cool, and pour over the melted chocolate.

7)   Sugar free apple pie

Ingredients:
- **5 apples + 1 to decorate**
- **170 grams of Greek yogurt**
- **150 grams of almonds**
- **2 eggs**
- **two tablespoons of coconut sugar**
- **a teaspoon of ground cinnamon**
- **a sachet of baking powder**
- **a pinch of salt**

Preheat the oven to 160 °. Grease and flour the mold. Put the eggs, yogurt, coconut sugar, peeled and coarsely cut apples, salt, yeast, cinnamon, and flour in a blender. Blend everything very well, collecting the finished mixture in the walls and blending again. Pour the mixture into the pan and decorate with thin apple slices. Bake for 50 minutes and, before turning out, do the toothpick test, which must come out dry. Remove the apple pie from the oven and let it rest for 10 minutes, then gently transfer it to a wire rack to cool. Serve your apple pie without sugar, and enjoy it!

8)   Caramelized pineapple

Ingredients:
- 1 fresh pineapple
- 1 teaspoon non-fat butter
- 2 tablespoons of coconut sugar
- a pinch of cinnamon

Clean the pineapple by removing its ends and peel with a sharp knife. Then cut it into regular slices. In a large pan melt the butter, lay the pineapple slices and brown them on both sides for about 5 minutes. Spread the sugar and cinnamon over and melt, turn the pineapple slices over and over until the sugar has turned into a thick, caramel brown. Turn off and serve!

9)   Fruit popsicles and Greek yogurt

Ingredients:
- 10 Strawberries
- 1 Kiwi
- 100 g Greek yogurt
- 50 ml Coconut milk
- 1 tablespoon agave syrup
- 1 vanilla bean

Wash and dry the strawberries. Remove the stalk and cut it into pieces, transfer them to a blender and reduce them to cream. Pour the blended strawberries into the appropriate popsicle molds and put them in the freezer to solidify for about half an hour. In this way, when you pour the other ingredients, they will not mix. In the meantime, put the Greek yogurt, coconut milk, and agave syrup in a bowl. Remove the seeds from the vanilla pod with the tip of a knife and add them to the cream. Mix the yogurt cream with a small whisk and place it in the fridge to cool. Peel the kiwi, cut it into pieces, and blend it. Pour the smoothie kiwi into the molds that you put in the freezer and solidify it for another half hour. Finally, pour the yogurt cream into the molds and insert the appropriate stick. Leave to cool for at least two hours.

10) Sugar-free meringues

Ingredients:
- **3 egg whites**
- **1 pinch of cream of tartar**
- **orange peel**
- **60 g of birch xylitol**

Reduce xylitol to powder with a food processor. Whip the egg whites with the addition of some cream of tartar. After about two minutes, add the xylitol and the peel of an orange (or lemon). Keep whipping until you get a soft meringue. With the help of a sac-à-poche, spread the meringue on baking paper at regular intervals. Bake at 90 ° C for 2 hours. Turn off the oven and let it dry overnight.

11) Sugar-free chocolate bombs
Ingredients:
- **500 g Light mascarpone**
- **300 g 75% dark chocolate**
- **300 g Cocoa paste**
- **2 tablespoons Agave syrup (or coconut sugar syrup)**

- **100 g chopped hazelnuts**
- **100 g Almond grains**
- **100 g Pistachio grains**
- **3 tbsp grated coconut**

Pour the two types of chopped chocolate into a glass bowl, melt the chocolate in a bain-marie or the microwave, provided they are low-powered so as not to burn the chocolate. Stir the chocolate occasionally while it melts. Once the chocolate has melted, add the agave syrup and mix well. At this point, add the mascarpone and incorporate it well with the help of a spatula. Cover the bowl with plastic wrap, put the mixture in the fridge to cool for half an hour. Spread the dried fruit and coconut in 4 soup plates. Take the hardened mixture in the fridge, and with the dampened hands, take a small portion and rotate it in your hands until you get a small ball. Place the praline in a tray and continue until the mixture is finished, wet your hands with fresh water. Put 4-5 pralines on the plate with the grain and rotate until the pralines are completely covered. Take them from the plate, compact the grains on the praline by dropping the excess. Place the covered praline on a baking tray and continue until the covered pralines are finished. Now your sugar-free chocolate pralines are ready. You can arrange them in a tray or on a large plate and put them in the fridge covered with plastic wrap or paper, where they will be kept for 5-6 days.

12) Granita

Ingredients:
- **400 ml Coconut milk**
- **a spoonful of Stevia powder (satin)**
- **200 g 70-85% dark chocolate**
- **50 ml coconut milk**
- **Mint (for garnish)**

Mix the Stevia coconut milk and melt it well. Pour the coconut milk into the ice cube molds and place in the freezer to freeze. When you want to serve the coconut milk granita, just melt the dark chocolate and mix it with the coconut milk. Pour the ice cubes into a blender and blend them until you get the granita. By giving intermittent strokes to not overheat it. Spread a nice spoonful of melted chocolate on the bottom of 4 bowls and pour over the granita. Garnish with fresh mint leaves and serve. Enjoy this delicious and fresh summer dessert!

Chapter 9: Sauces & Condiments

1) Guacamole

Ingredients:
- **Ripe avocado 1**
- **Green hot pepper 1**
- **Auburn tomatoes 1**
- **Extra virgin olive oil 20 g**
- **Lime juice 10 g**
- **Shallot 10 g**
- **Black pepper 1 pinch**
- **Salt up to a pinch**

Start by cutting the avocado in half lengthwise, remove the core, and extract the pulp. Put everything in a bowl. Cut the lime in half and extract the juice, to be poured over the avocado pulp. Then season with salt and pepper, and mash the pulp with a fork. Set aside, then clean and finely chop the shallot, then wash, dry, and slice the tomato and cut into cubes. Then tick the chili, remove its seeds and cut it into strips, then diced. Add everything to the bowl with the crushed avocado pulp. Add the oil, mix, and season again with salt and pepper if necessary. Your guacamole sauce is ready to be enjoyed!

2) Pistachio pesto

Ingredients:
- **Unsalted unsalted pistachios (shelled) 200 g**
- **Grated cheese 35 g**

- ½ lemon zest
- ½ clove garlic
- Extra virgin olive oil 100 ml
- Water 100 ml
- Basil 3 leaves
- Salt to taste
- Black pepper to taste

Place a pot full of water on the fire, bring it to the boil, pour the shelled pistachios, and cook for about 5 minutes. Remove the pistachio peel and collect them in a bowl. Transfer the pistachios to a mixer, pour the olive oil, grated cheese, basil leaves, lemon zest of half a lemon, and half a clove of garlic. Operate the blades for a few moments, pour the water, salt, pepper, and operate the blades again, whisk the mixture until obtaining a homogenous cream.

3) Rocket pesto

Ingredients:
- 100 g rocket already cleaned
- 50 g of shelled and toasted walnuts
- 50 g of grated pecorino cheese
- 50 g of grated Parmesan cheese
- 1 clove of garlic
- extra virgin olive oil
- salt
- pepper

To prepare the arugula pesto, collect all the ingredients in the mixing bowl or a common blender. Blend by adding oil flush from the hole on the lid and stirring occasionally.

Set the times according to the desired consistency: you will still need to obtain a homogeneous cream. Once ready you can use the rocket pesto immediately, to season the pasta diluting it with a little cooking water, or you can transfer it to a hermetically sealed glass container, cover it with a veil of oil and put it in the refrigerator, where it will be kept for a couple of days.

4) Tuna sauce

Ingredients:
- 100 g of tuna in oil
- 50 g of pickled capers
- 2 anchovies
- 1 hard yolk
- 1/2 lemon juice
- 1 glass of extra virgin olive oil
- salt
- pepper

Start chopping the tuna well drained from the oil and collect it in the mixing bowl together with the rinsed and squeezed capers, the dehydrated anchovies, and the hard-boiled egg yolk. Soften the dough with a few tablespoons of oil and operate the appliance with short clicks. Gradually add the rest of the oil and blend for a few seconds until the desired density is obtained. Add the lemon juice filtered through a strainer and mix very well. Taste and, if necessary, adjust salt and pepper. Let it sit for 10 minutes. If the sauce is too thick, dilute it with a little oil. Then pour the tuna sauce in a gravy boat or serving bowl and serve.

5) Hollandaise sauce

Ingredients:
- 3 eggs
- 30 g of lemon juice
- salt
- pepper

- **150 g of vegetable butter**
- **2 spoons of water**

Put the water on the fire in a large enough saucepan to house another in a water bath. In the smallest pan, collect the yolks, the two spoons of cold water and the salt, and with the help of a whisk, work them for about 10 minutes, until they have reached the consistency of thick cream. In the meantime, melt the butter and start adding it to the sauce, little by little, flush. Keep beating with the whisk. Be careful that the water in the water bath does not reach a boil, and it would risk making the sauce go crazy. When the sauce thickens, add the lemon, a pinch of pepper, and season with salt. The result must be creamy. If the hollandaise sauce has thickened excessively, add a few drops of warm water. If you do not serve the sauce immediately, keep it hot in a double boiler, do not heat it on the fire. Again, the water in the water bath should not be too hot. Bring the hollandaise sauce to the table in a sauceboat.

6)   Tzatziki

Ingredients:
- **250 g of Greek yogurt**
- **1 cucumber**
- **2 teaspoons of chopped dill**
- **1 teaspoon vinegar**
- **1 clove of garlic**
- **salt**
- **extra virgin olive oil**

Clean and finely chop the garlic. Wash the cucumber well and without peeling it, finely chop it, add salt and drain it. Pour the yogurt into a bowl, add the squeezed cucumber, the chopped dill and garlic, the vinegar and season with salt. Mix everything and serve, seasoning the surface with extra virgin olive oil.

7)   Bernese sauce

Ingredients:

- **200 g of melted fat-free butter**
- **1 dl of vinegar**
- **4 shallots**
- **2 tablespoons of fresh tarragon**
- **3 yolks**
- **lemon juice**
- **1 pinch of cayenne pepper**
- **Salt**

In a steel saucepan, pour the vinegar, add the chopped shallots, and half the tarragon, salt. Let the liquid reduce to more than half. Remove from the heat, filter the remaining vinegar by applying light pressure and let it cool. In a saucepan, start whipping the yolks with the electric whisk, adding the infusion of vinegar and shallots flush. When the mixture becomes frothy, put it in a water bath (the water must be already warm), always continuing to mount. When the cream appears well whipped, add the melted butter, little by little, working with the whisk until the mixture has reached a creamy, smooth and homogeneous consistency. Transfer the sauce to a bowl, adjust it with pepper, complete with the remaining tarragon and, taste, with a few drops of lemon juice.

8)   Almond milk mayonnaise

Ingredients:
- **500 g unsweetened almond milk**
- **175 g of extra virgin olive oil**
- **juice and zest of 1/2 lemon**
- **salt**

Start by simmering the almond milk until its volume is reduced by 50%. Let it cool down to room temperature. Strain the milk and pour it into a container. Add the lemon juice and a pinch of salt. Emulsify with an immersion blender, pouring the oil flush, until a thick and frothy mayonnaise is obtained. For an even fresher flavor, add the grated lemon zest.

9)   Vegan hazelnut cream

Ingredients:
- **100 g of toasted hazelnuts**
- **150 g of 75% dark chocolate**
- **150 g of 85% dark chocolate**
- **150 g of coconut sugar**
- **150 g of soy milk**
- **80 g of corn seed oil**

Pour the hazelnuts into a mixer and blend until a very fine mixture is obtained. Cut the dark chocolate into coarse flakes and place them in the glass of the immersion blender. Heat the soy milk and pour it boiling over the chocolate, stirring to melt it. Then blend to even out the mixture. Add the sugar and the chopped hazelnuts, mix with a spatula, and whisk for a long time to homogenize everything. Finally, add the oil dose and blend it again. With the help of a spatula, pour the cream into one or more jars, cap, and keep cool.

10) Green sauce

Ingredients:

- **Anchovies in oil fillets 3**
- **2 cloves garlic**
- **Parsley 120 g**
- **Capers in salt 1 tbsp**
- **Hard yolks 2**
- **White wine vinegar 50 g**
- **Wholemeal stale bread (only the crumb) 80 g**
- **Extra virgin olive oil 150 g**
- **Black pepper to taste**
- **Salt to taste**

Put the water to heat in a pan, and as soon as the water is boiling, immerse the eggs that will have to be covered with water and cook them for about 8-9 minutes, then let them cool for a few moments before peeling them. Finally, sift the yolks into a bowl. Then, remove the crust of the bread, cut the crumb into pieces, and pour it into a bowl with the vinegar. Soak for about ten minutes. Meanwhile, peel, divide the garlic in half. Desalinate the capers by rinsing them under running water and mince them together with the garlic and anchovies; They pass the blade over the mince to crush it well to obtain a well-mixed pasta you will pour into the bowl with the yolk. Squeeze the crumb with your hands and put it in the bowl. Finally, finely chop the parsley leaves, wash and dry, and pour them into the bowl together with a pinch of salt and pepper. Mix thoroughly and sprinkle with extra virgin olive oil. Let it sit at room temperature for a couple

of hours, and your green sauce is ready to accompany
your favorite dishes, from boiled fish to fish to croutons!

11) Spreadable cream without sugar

Ingredients:
- **450 g Toasted hazelnuts**
- **1 tablespoon Stevia (or 2 of coconut sugar)**
- **40 g Bitter cocoa powder**
- **1 tablespoon seed oil**

Pour the hazelnuts into the blender, blend them at maximum power for about 5 minutes, until a thick cream is obtained. Collect the cream on the edges with a spatula and blend again for a minute. Pour the stevia and cocoa over the hazelnut cream and blend again. Collect the mixture again and pour in the oil, blend again for 30 seconds. Pour the sugar-free spreadable cream into a jar, or several small, sterilized jars and close with the cap. Place the spreadable cream in the fridge, cooling and firming.

12) Sugar free pastry cream

Ingredients:

- **1/2 l Partially skimmed milk**
- **2 eggs**
- **1 tablespoon coconut flour**
- **2 teaspoons Stevia**
- **1/2 vanilla bean**
- **1 orange zest (or lemon)**
- **1 pinch of salt**

Separate the yolks from the whites and whisk them. Pour the yolks into a saucepan, add the stevia and the flour and dilute. Pour the milk slowly and mix well. Flavor the milk with the seeds from the vanilla pod, the orange zest, and the salt. Place the saucepan on the heat, add the whipped egg whites and, constantly stirring, bring to a light boil until a thick and velvety custard is obtained. Remove from the heat, remove the peel of the citrus fruit of your choice, and cover with a sheet of film, until it cools. Now your sugar-free custard is ready to be enjoyed!

Conclusion

PCOS is a disorder that compromises a woman's quality of life due to the presence of male hormones. Over time, this condition can lead to changes in the physical appearance of a woman, which causes emotional distress and depressive forms. PCOS is one of the most common obstacles for all women who want to get pregnant. The characteristic of polycystic ovary syndrome is filling with microscopic fluid-filled cysts, which prevent follicles from producing ovulation during the ovulation phase. PCOS per se is not life-threatening but, if neglected for a long time, can lead to even serious complications such as type 2 diabetes and Endometrial cancer. Although many women become aware of this syndrome only when they wish to become pregnant, it is advisable to contact your doctor immediately to give you the right indications and treatments to deal with this disorder.